THE STRENGTH COACH

RECOVERY AND THE HANGOVER SYNDROME

CONTAINING EXTRACTS FROM:

THE STRENGTH COACH
TRAINING TECHNIQUES AND METHODS

THE STRENGTH COACH
COACHING AND MOTIVATING POWERLIFTERS

THE STRENGTH COACH
THE KEYS TO SUCCESSFUL STRENGTH TRAINING

BY: *PAUL KERRIDGE*

WARNING

This booklet contains advice on training techniques used by elite powerlifters and strength athletes. The methods and procedures may be dangerous if not performed correctly and with competent assistance. The explanations and all the advice given in this book are for your personal use entirely at your own risk and this book is made available only on the condition that the reader accepts this condition completely. As with any exercise regime, it's the participating individual's responsibility to ensure they are not at any specific or general risk in undertaking a weight training strength development programme.

....

ONE OF THE STRENGTH COACH SERIES OF BOOKS AND INFORMATION BOOKLETS PUBLISHED BY KERRIDGE SPORTS PUBLICATIONS 2015

EDITION – 4   July 2024

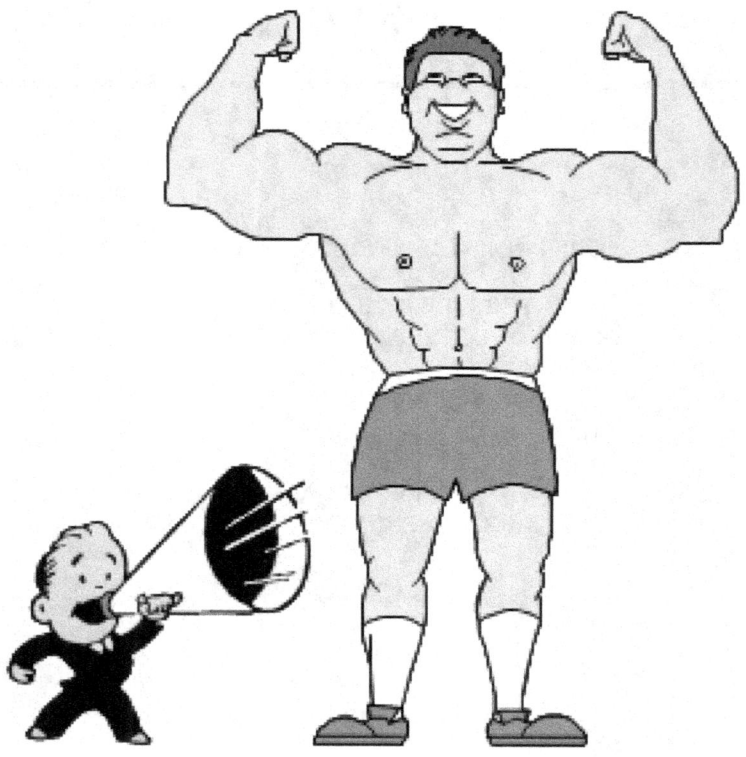

FOREWORD BY THE AUTHOR

After spending over half a century training with weights, I can say with some authority that I've made all the mistakes its been possible to make. Luckily I've learnt a thing or two along the way, and one particular issue stands out above all others from my research and practical experience. This is recovery in general, and specifically the lack of recovery from poorly designed programmes that apply repeated stress on muscles before they have had time to adapt. Repeated sessions within a short timescale is one obvious cause, but a key element is simply incorrect exercise selection. This booklet explains in detail how getting this wrong can delay or ruin any prospect of strength development and muscle increase. In my opinion workout design remains a major problem for those looking to develop, often leading to stagnation and injury. I call this lack of recovery the 'hangover syndrome'. Recovery hangovers play a significant part in the build-up of injuries in any activity or sport where resistance training is a part of the development programme. Knowledge is key for developing any area of human activity and without it so much effort and energy is simply wasted, and strength training is no exception. Until I fully understood this relationship between training and recovery I had personally used and even recommended programmes that were plagued by serious recovery problems. It's embarrassing when I think about it now! After many years of research and coaching I can now show you how poor recovery inhibits your progress, but more importantly how you can overcome the hidden hangovers in any workout plan. Get it right and the results are dramatic from a few simple changes to your exercise routine. Reading this booklet will ensure you understand the 'hangover syndrome' completely enabling you to review any programme to eliminate recovery issues. Hangovers appear in almost all training plans I review, usually without the author or coach understanding why. The difference between a well organised hangover free plan will become visible once you understand the underlying key principles. I have included a simple process to check programmes for yourself as well as several real case reviews to demonstrate how to do it. Learn how to examine training programmes with new knowledge to eliminate this hidden performance limiting menace.

Paul Kerridge

1. STRENGTH AND MUSCLE DEVELOPMENT FACTORS

Before getting into the detailed issues around recovery I will briefly cover the basics that apply to physical development, both muscular and neurological. Understanding these issues will ensure you appreciate why some training parameters are critical, and others less so. Your progress will be significantly accelerated with the right combination of training and recovery, however if you get it wrong progress will be slowed or impeded altogether. This first chapter summarises the most important factors you should be aware of, so lets start.

1.1 Central nervous system (CNS) adaptation for muscle motor unit recruitment rate.

The recruitment rate refers to the speed at which you can muster a strong contraction of a muscle. When your brain decides to make any movement there is a delay before the muscles fully contract, and this can be improved with the right training. Adaptions from dynamic (speed) training improve this speed to maximum contraction. A faster time to maximum contraction strength improves applied momentum to the body during a sporting movement or a weight used in exercise giving the athlete an advantage. Field strength athletes and Olympic lifters who need to produce explosive force in minimal time value this type of strength improvement training above all others. It's developed with what is generally called 'power' or 'dynamic' training. Explosive strength developed in this way assists the overall capability of any sportsman or athlete.

1.2 CNS adaptation for neurological coordination of muscles in a movement.

Coordination is a acquired skill. The Central Nervous System must learn to coordinate all the muscles used for any movement including those acting as fixing or supporting muscles. Practice using thousands of repetitions embed muscle coordination patterns in the brain improving mechanical efficiency, confidence and performance. All new movements or activities take time to cultivate efficiency. This is one reason why beginners to weight training make very rapid progress as they become accustomed to unfamiliar movements and exercises. Adaptation for efficiency may take as many as 10,000 repetitions to become fully embedded and proficient.

1.3 CNS adaptation for synchronous rather than asynchronous motor unit recruitment.

All skeletal muscles contain bundles of fibres grouped in units called motor units, each with a single nerve attachment for firing the contraction. The motor unit can only be on or off, nothing in between other than the pulse rate of firing. Increments in applied strength come from more or less bundles being fired and at a higher pulse rate. The brain learns how to coordinate the firing of these separate motor units to perform movements at varied contraction strength. Some motor units are very small allowing delicate contractions for fine movements while others are large to allow firm contractions for greater strength. When undertaking most normal low intensity activity the CNS shares the load by alternating the contraction of motor units. Alternating these motor units allow some to rest and recover while others take the load. This alternating process is called asynchronous activation which extends the total endurance of a muscle allowing for activities such as walking or running to be maintained for hours. However, with intense contractions above 50% of a muscle's contraction capability the sharing of the load between motor units becomes limited and above 80% of single contraction strength (1RM) such sharing becomes impossible. This is why repetition capability decreases with increasing resistance load. Under normal circumstances the CNS is used to activate muscles in the sharing asynchronous mode as most people rarely, if ever have to apply a maximum singular muscular effort to any task. Consequently, the CNS in untrained individuals is inefficient when it comes to applying maximum strength and it has to learn how to activate a high percentage of muscle motor units in synchronous mode efficiently to produce greater strength. This aspect of developing strength is a major contributor to early performance improvement in untrained individuals.

1.4 CNS adaptation to Golgi and Spindle organs.

These organs are present in all major muscles and their tendons. They sense tension, rotational position of the skeleton joints and the speed of contraction. Information from these organs is fed into the CNS constantly and feedback from any movement allows the brain to learn how to apply muscle contractions to achieve the desired position and strength of movement. However, they also signal warnings to limit the contractions or increase the tension in an opposing muscle as a protective mechanism avoiding over extending a joint or tearing a muscle. Heavy training reduces the involuntary impact of this protective mechanism allowing greater contraction, and hence applied strength.

1.5 Improved psychological focus, commitment and motivation.

Improving mental focus and commitment to an action enables a far greater voluntary muscle contraction to take place. Mental focus makes a huge difference to lifting a weight and even experienced lifters can gain from appropriate stimulation techniques. A casual approach will always result in a poor performance, so developing good mental focus techniques is an important part of strength training development.

1.6 Improved anatomical positioning and technique.

The grip, stance, foot position and various other anatomical and technique changes may make a significant contribution to the outcome when lifting heavy weights or applying strength to any sporting activity. Beginners to any sport soon make progress through developing better technique and anatomical positioning.

1.7 Improved muscle efficiency from greater contraction chemical storage and blood flow.

Any muscle becomes more efficient through better blood flow, hydration and the greater storage of glycogen and creatine as well as several other important chemicals. With improved efficiency muscles are able to operate faster, longer and recover quicker between sets and after the workout. Better recovery allows a greater frequency of training and hence faster long term development. Muscle efficiency is improved with consistent training over long periods.

1.8 Increased muscle size from greater protein myosin/actin cross-links.

Muscles grow in two ways, through increased vascular capacity and fluid in and surrounding the muscle as well as actual hypertrophy of individual muscle fibres. Additional protein cross-links are laid down following intense contractions during the super compensation stage as a means to protect the muscle from further stress. This adaptation takes time and body resources to accomplish and cannot be rushed. The process is complicated and dependant on diet and rest. In many ways this issue is the most important for long term development of strength and muscle size.

2. THE MUSCULAR DEVELOPMENT CYCLE

Improvement in muscular performance and size is driven by the central nervous system and hormonal signals generated by muscular stress. Long term development ultimately relies on the muscle's physical contraction capacity from growth, efficiency and CNS learning. Strength athletes get bigger over time whether intended or not due to the growth in vascular capacity and the hypertrophy of the exercised muscles. While bodybuilders generally train entirely differently to gain size, they also grow in strength. The goals may be different, but the outcomes from the often differing regimes have very obvious similarities. Designing training plans with specific goals in mind is essential, you would not train for a marathon by swimming or discus throwing just as you would not train for a powerlifting competition by running long distance. Anyone who trains with weights or resistance share the common factors of growth and strength gains in varying degrees from such training. However, recovery is the most often overlooked issue in many training plans. This booklet explains the relevant recovery issues experienced while developing muscles primarily used to increase strength and a more efficient contraction capacity. However, growth in muscular size will inevitably follow strength improvements. Before we can discuss recovery issues we need to consider what strength athletes or bodybuilders actually do to train themselves to get stronger and bigger. This we call the muscular development cycle.

To achieve muscular growth, or strength improvement some training process has to occur. While there are many training alternatives to achieve this, ultimately they are all variations on a simple theme. The muscles, as well as the central nervous system need an adequate stimulus or stress followed by time to recover fully before repeating the cycle. Following recovery to pre-stress normality the CNS and hormonal signals within the muscles themselves stimulate a small additional capacity to help avoid a similar stress putting the body at risk. The added capacity is mainly a small increase in protein links on the stressed muscle fibres, but also includes CNS learning to recognise and embed nerve contraction patterns, and how best they are applied. This added capacity of the muscles and CNS is called super compensation and it's a natural consequence of allowing the body to recover fully and adapt. **Fig.1** represents this cyclic process. After an adequate training stimulus the body as a whole moves into a recovery phase where localised and systemic processes recuperate depleted chemicals, remove waste products and start to repair damaged tissues. The process continues with the CNS driving super compensation, adding a small increment in strength from muscular hypertrophy. This adaptation results in the muscles capacity to repeat a similar stress with less injury and is a common biological process allowing all mammals and many other animals to slowly adapt to their environment in order to survive. A simple visible example is the adaptation process when handling rough or heavy objects. Calluses develop to protect the skin from further stress. Clearly, if the abrasion is too

Fig.1

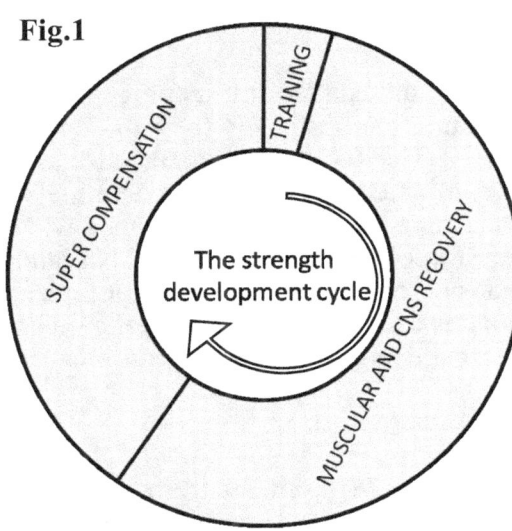

extreme the skin will break and injury occurs, conversely, if the abrasion is low the skin has no need to develop calluses and no adaptation occurs. This simple example often quoted in training books highlights an important biological lesson that we need to consider when strength training. Getting stronger without injury is just like developing calluses without blisters. Light exercise does not produce the stimulus required, whereas excessive heavy stress is likely to injure and prevent

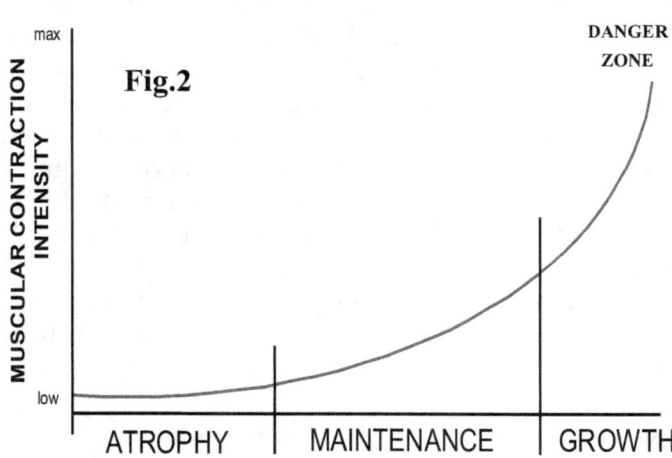

super compensation. What's needed is an appropriate level of training stress followed by enough rest for the biological recovery, adaptation and super compensation to occur. **Fig.2** shows how differing levels of muscular stress impact on the body. The 'use it or lose it' principle applies and to grow you need an abnormal stress that does not injure. Going about your normal daily routine simply maintains your existing muscle size. Adaptation to an external influence underpins the whole concept of training to develop and improve size or strength, but it's not a simple process. In fact, the biological recovery and adaptation process is both complex and highly dependent on several specific systems that combine to deliver the full recovery and super compensation effect. Let's consider what actually needs to recover in a little detail in the following chapter.

3. KEY ELEMENTS OF THE RECOVERY PROCESS

The recovery and any subsequent adaptation from physical training activity is complex and varies with the type of exercise employed, its intensity, duration and external influences such as environment and diet. In this chapter I will summarise all the important issues involved.

Following a training event there are a number of body functions, maintenance and support systems that kick into action. These may be localised or systemic in nature, but ultimately they all depend on internal systems, diet and lifestyle to complete successfully. The fuels, hormones and waste products that are depleted or created must be replaced or eliminated before damaged tissue is repaired to regain equilibrium. In addition, more resources and time are required to enhance what previously existed, in a word, 'development'. Then, often forgotten there are the CNS and psychological elements of recovery that also need to be considered. Some of these biological activities recover to normal levels quickly in seconds and minutes after exercise, others take much longer. The following section is a discussion regarding these post exercise recovery requirements. It starts with the most basic of all, breathing and oxygen.

3.1 Oxygen and lactate.

The most recognisable additional demand and consequent recovery requirement from strenuous exercise is oxygen uptake. During, and following a high stress demand on the body the heart rate and respiration are elevated to provide additional oxygen for muscular action. This is largely related to aerobic activity, but still occurs with anaerobic short bursts of activity such a lifting a heavy weight if the effort is intense enough. The demand for greater oxygen from breathing usually subsides quickly in seconds after short bursts of anaerobic exercise, such as after a heavy deadlift, but this may last for several minutes following highly stressful aerobic activity like a run at near maximum capacity. While oxygen levels and respiration recover very quickly from a short burst of anaerobic activity with very minor ongoing recovery of any consequence, after any prolonged intense exercise for more than a few minutes a deficit known as an oxygen debt will have been built, and like any debt it has to be repaid. This debt is a result of low oxygen available in the blood around the muscles forcing the anaerobic use of glycogen and the consequent creation of lactic acid as a means to maintain contractions during this immediate shortage. The lactic acid becomes lactate in the blood which accumulates if the exercise or stress is maintained during this ongoing shortage of oxygen. Lactate has to be cleared after exercise which involves an ongoing increased uptake of oxygen to resolve. The oxygen lactate topic has been studied extensively and the generic graph in **Fig.3** shows the generation of an oxygen debt at the start of a moderately

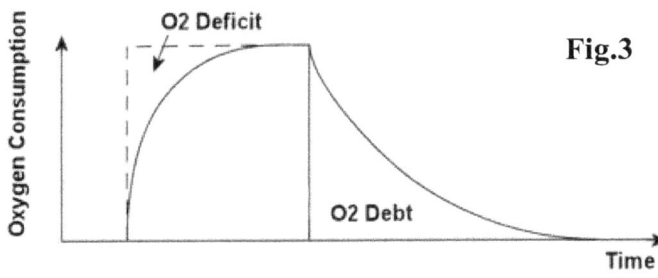

intense exercise followed by a plateau where the demand is matched by intake if the activity level is within the individuals capacity to maintain. The plateau at the top of the graph may extend considerably in the case of long distance runners or cyclists performing comfortably within their current capacity for long periods. After the activity, respiration may appear to quickly return to normal, but oxygen uptake remains high before decreasing slowly towards normal resting levels. During this post exercise period the extra oxygen is used to repay the debt in conjunction with the liver by removal or conversion of the lactic acid back to blood glucose. The repayment duration can extend to 24 hours or more in extreme cases, but for most aerobic training situations it will return to normal levels in several hours. Weight training consisting of short duration sets produces little oxygen debt with a correspondingly low recovery requirement. As a rule of thumb, if an exercise leaves you breathing heavily then some oxygen debt has been introduced requiring recovery, and the longer the heavy breathing period the larger the likely debt and the recovery period. Aerobic training improves the capacity of the body to intake oxygen to meet demand which is clearly observed as individuals get fitter aerobically. For example, if you consider an individual at the start of a jogging programme to several weeks later. At first they will become breathless very quickly at low run speeds, but as the training improves their lung capacity and corresponding 'fitness' they will be capable of jogging further or faster before this breathlessness becomes an issue. Such improvement has a direct impact on the oxygen debt initially generated and the following repayment recovery period.

Now, consider this, an individual training for strength may want to perform three sets of squats using 80% of their 1RM after a warm-up as part of their routine. The exertion from such a routine will likely push them into the heavy breathing lactic acid generation zone. Then, they have to get fired up for the next two sets. Usually such training will include inter set rest periods of up to 5 minutes or even more. Despite such long rests, if the oxygen debt and blood lactic has not been cleared they will start subsequent sets at a disadvantage compared to their initial condition. The following sets may then go on to add to the oxygen debt and blood lactic levels detracting from potential maximum performance. Consequently, it makes sense for anyone who trains with weights using moderate to high intensity to ensure they take long rests between sets and consider their aerobic fitness as a means to reduce such oxygen debt and improve blood lactate clearance. Improving these processes will aid ongoing training performance and hence long term development.

Lets now consider the specific issue of Lactate. Lactic acid builds up from the anaerobic muscular use of glycogen during highly intense exercise as already mentioned or when aerobic exercise pushes the oxygen requirements beyond current oxygen intake capacity. The effect of lactic build up presents itself as pain and burning in the exercised muscles, and sometimes the chest. It can cause nausea when pushed to the limit using a high repetition range for an individual exercise set, or from multiple sets or circuit training performed with low inter-set rests such as HIT training. My old boxing coach would not be happy unless at least one of us in the squad was throwing up after a hard fitness session, but that's another very long story.

The point at which lactate becomes a problem may be relatively quick where anaerobic stress during the lack of oxygen is high, such as from 12 heavy repetitions of squats or from multiple sets with short rests. However, it's always an issue with higher repetitions for any single exercise set where heavy breathing is generated. The affect is notable with bodybuilders using drop or rest pause sets and individuals performing circuit fitness training. The science is complex and is usually explained as two interacting parameters, the lactate build up point, and the lactate clearance capacity. The good news is that both of these parameters may be improved with appropriate training. While lactate build up is not the sole reason for muscular fatigue it does play an important part. For example, an individual starting an exercise programme may be able to reach 50 repetitions for an exercise with a relatively light 10 kilos before experiencing a high lactic build up in the exercised muscles forcing them to stop. This may also occur doing just 12 repetitions with the same exercise at 20 kilos over three sets with short rests. Some time later after a period of appropriate training the same individual may be able to reach 70 repetitions with 10 kilos or 6 sets of 12 repetitions with 20 kilos before experiencing the pain of excessive lactate. In this case the individual will have improved both their mental capacity to keep going while in pain, as well as

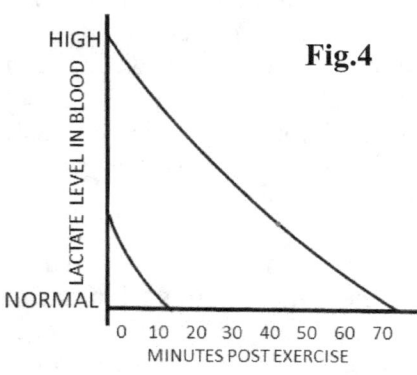

Fig.4

having improved the lactate build up point and clearance rate. The beginning where build up starts to create problems varies greatly with individuals and their conditioning. Improving tolerance to this build up, as well as the clearance rate improving from training has a direct impact on inter-set and post exercise session recovery. While the recovery time post exercise cannot be directly defined due to the great variability between individuals and their conditioning, we know that the lactate level in the blood returns to normal following high levels in healthy people within 1-2 hours and much faster from lower stress induced levels. **Fig.4** shows a generic model of this clearance derived from several notable medical experiments.

With training, the body improves the build up point and tolerance to the affect allowing a greater continued performance before having to stop exercising and a faster clearance rate allowing the individual to recover greater muscle function between exercise sets or sessions. Several recent medical studies reveal a considerable improvement in recovery time where light activity is undertaken compared to passive rest both between sets and in later recovery periods.

While training improvements in lactic tolerance and clearance are not considered as part of the classic strength gain and hypertrophy super compensation process, it obviously impacts on the ability of an individual to continue and repeat an exercise. Hence, the loading capacity during a session for any individual may be increased having developed better lactate tolerance and clearance. Using the example above, if the individual after some training is able to perform 6 sets with 20 kilos rather than the previous 3 due to improved tolerance and clearance rates, then the greater training load will likely increase hypertrophy compensation from added muscular micro-damage, assuming full muscular recovery is allowed following the session. In addition, the confidence and mental strength improvement from experiencing and overcoming the desire to stop should not be underestimated. Consequently, the effect of improving lactate handling must be considered as part of the overall training affect and recovery.

We know that high repetition exercise is not an effective method to develop pure strength as many studies have shown lower repetitions with heavier weights to be far more effective. So, most trainees interested in pure strength development rarely venture into the high lactic generation zone. However, some training programmes, particularly for body building that use higher repetitions and multiple sets will create far more lactic acid. Improving lactic tolerance and recovery from such programmes contributes to improving general aerobic fitness and mental strength although this is not considered as a primary recovery issue for hypertrophy. The two issues of oxygen and lactate are clearly entwined making the aerobic fitness of any athlete, regardless of their aims of considerable importance in ongoing training capacity, and hence potential progressive development.

3.2 Hydration.
The evidence from many medical studies reveals the importance of hydration for all athletes and sportsmen for both performance and recovery. Poor hydration results in lower performance in aerobic and anaerobic muscle action and de-hydration extends recovery. Any training event is improved by starting fully hydrated where the urine is virtually clear, followed by regular topping up to maintain hydration during and post exercise. Lets look at this important issue in some detail.

If you're normally a little dehydrated, which is the base state for most people, correct hydration can improve your best single squat by 5%. That's a fact supported by sports science studies. When did you last gain that much so easily on any of your best lifts? The benefit of full hydration depends on your normal hydration and for some individuals who are dehydrated most of the time the potential is considerable. For sports that involve endurance a 20% gain in performance is not uncommon from correcting poor hydration. Despite many scientific studies proving this advantage its importance is rarely discussed outside of endurance sports circles in the UK. Many coaches know the importance of good hydration without understanding the full potential loss of performance, thinking it's only relevant in hot climates. There are few deaths or heat strokes in the UK due to sports dehydration, but go to Australia, Spain or Africa and coaches have a different perspective entirely. They're acutely aware of the serious problems that occur if an athlete doesn't take care to maintain hydration. In a hot climate this is a key topic for any sport and the effects are very clear if you get it wrong. For example, a 100kg individual playing rugby or football in a warm climate can lose 4-6% of their bodyweight in sweat during a match. That's up to 6 kilograms! A classic and very visual example of dehydration in practice is often seen on the TV when a football match in the summer goes into extra time. The players stop for that few minutes, then like a growing plague they all begin dropping to the ground grasping their calves and legs as cramp takes hold. Cramps are a clear indication of dehydration and may last a few seconds or become extended to 15 minutes or more in severe cases. It's common for cramps to occur repeatedly in a muscle group over a period of hours, often overnight as the body becomes dehydrated. The reason is mainly a chemical imbalance between the sodium and potassium electrolyte fluid within the muscle due to sweating which expels sodium far more than any other electrolyte. This fact raises an important issue regarding recovery and re-hydration. Sports and exercise in hot weather can cause excessive fluid loss via perspiration and sweat is not just water. It contains salts, mostly as sodium and a little potassium and some other minerals in micro amounts. The combination of losing both fluid and electrolytes through sweating can increase heart rate, raise the body temperature and affect performance and recovery substantially.

Chronic volume depletion of body fluids from diuretics (medicines that promote urination) can mimic this dehydration without any excessive sweating during exercise. This is a known problem with bodybuilders who often lower their body fluid to dangerous levels before a show. It's also a common problem with athletes where they deliberately restrict water intake to achieve a body weight category such as in powerlifting and boxing. While the average male may happily survive on one gram of sodium chloride (table salt) per day normally provided by diet, there is a tendency these days for people to avoid salt as a health issue as it's linked to high blood pressure from water retention. A conundrum indeed! So, maintaining a high level of hydration where salt intake is low can become a problem requiring some additional salts added to the water being used to re-hydrate. Personally, I use a product called 'lowsalt' which is a mixture of sodium and potassium salts aimed at reducing sodium intake while providing that salty taste to food. It's a perfect substitute in small amounts for over the counter electrolyte replacement salts for electrolyte balance and replacement. Checking your hydration is easy using the urine colour test reference chart in **Fig.5**.

1	CLEAR **Fig.5**
2	LIGHT WHITE WINE COLOUR
3	WHITE WINE COLOUR
4	LIGHT YELLOW WINE COLOUR
5	DARK YELLOW
6	DARK YELLOW /LIGHT BROWN
7	LIGHT—DARK BROWN
8	DARK BROWN/GREEN

A full colour chart is available on the internet. Check by looking at the results of your pee in the toilet and add one level due to the dilution from the water in the pan, or for more accurate assessments take a small urine sample in a clear container and compare it to the urine dehydration chart against a white background. It's important to note that the effects of dehydration may take several hours to show in urine colour, so if you sweat a lot during an activity this may not show up for a while. The lighter the colour the better the hydration result. Colour ratings of 1, 2 or 3 are considered as well hydrated (Armstrong, 2000) with the deepening yellow 4 indicating a 2-3% dehydration. Based on the result, changes in fluid intake should be made. However, if the urine is totally clear you may be over hydrated and taking in too much fluid which can be counterproductive, and in severe cases dangerous if not accompanied by added electrolytes as mentioned above.

The one sure way to ensure you're fully hydrated before an event or workout is to start drinking water three hours beforehand every half hour until your pee runs nearly clear. This sort of routine is often undertaken by long distance runners before an event as the small regular amounts avoid any stomach bloating.

3.3 The specific effects on strength from dehydration.
Muscles contain around 70% of water by volume and most of the processes that allow our bodies to function rely on water (via blood) bourn chemicals. Adverse effects on performance occur with as little as a 1% reduction in bodyweight from optimal hydration, and most people are in this state or worse almost permanently.   The effect on endurance sports is well documented, but the affect on intense anaerobic exercise like weightlifting and powerlifting is far less understood in the sporting community. Fortunately one reliable study compared the strength at near 1RM performance for weightlifters. This medical study looked at the effects of partial dehydration on near maximum squats. They compared groups of athletes who were deliberately dehydrated with a control group with hydration managed at 100% throughout the study period. Two particular conclusions were found to be of importance.

1. The dehydrated group all reported greater levels of delayed onset muscle soreness (DOMS) following training sessions compared to the fully hydrated athletes. While the data on DOMS was subjective the results were significant. If training is carried out while partially dehydrated there will be a higher incidence of muscle damage and greater DOMS. This is an important issue for strength athletes as the super compensation gains will be delayed further due to the additional clearing of all damaged protein links within the muscle fibres. We know full recovery won't happen until the DOMS has been cleared and muscle re-synthesis completed. The conclusion must be that remaining fully hydrated during and post training reduces muscle micro stresses and accordingly must reduce the time for optimal recovery.

2. Dehydration was shown to impact directly on strength as powerlifters or weightlifters would relate, i.e. the near 1RM   results. The study used the squat as the test exercise with dehydration levels of -2.5% and -5% measured as temporary weight loss through sweating. This resulted in an average 1RM strength loss of 1.7% and 3.35% respectively.
   This may not sound like a large loss, but at competitions I have seen the totals of the three powerlifting exercises between first and third place varying by as little as 10 kilograms. I personally won the British three lift powerlifting competition only 2.5 kilograms ahead of the Scottish champion. That difference was only 2.7% of my body weight, so a small change

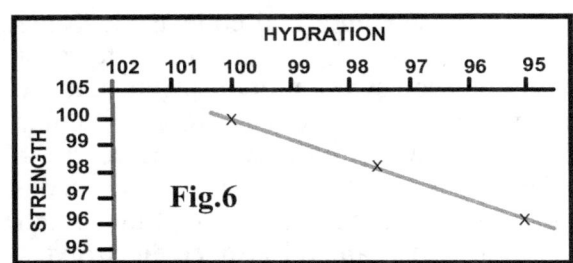

Fig.6

in hydration at the limits in competition can make all the difference. The results from the medical study are shown on the graph in **Fig.6** and you can see a direct and distinct correlation between hydration and muscular strength. The science is confirmed in practice when powerlifters dehydrate to make a weight limit in competition.

These lifters almost always report a disappointing competition result where weights lifted in the gym become difficult or impossible. In powerlifting a 3.35% loss of strength is enough to create a very serious problem.

A number of other notable studies have been conducted and the results of some are shown in **Fig.7.**

REFERANCE	%BW LOSS	STRENGTH	
Geenleaf 1967	-3%	0	**Fig.7**
Bosco 1968	-3%	-11%	
Houston 1981	-8%	-11%	
Webster 1990	-7%	-5%	
Montain 1998	-4%	0	
Schoffstall 2001	-1.5%	-6%	

Unfortunately the definition of strength is dubious in some of these medical studies and the results are outrageously variable. However, the results shown in **Fig.6** are reliable and are relevant to strength sports and powerlifting, in addition they are conservative and average with unusual results discarded as it's common practice in controlled medical studies to discard very high or very low results as anomalies. But, it's entirely possible that 'Bosco' in 1968 who showed a huge 11% drop in performance from a 3% dehydration could apply to you as an individual. That's a sobering thought for your next heavy gym session or your squat and deadlift preparation for a competition!

The vital take out from all this information is that hydration is critical for both peak performance and minimising your recovery whatever sport or activity you pursue. Recovery will vary with the amount of de-hydration and the type and volume of fluid intake post exercise. It's not achieved quickly and a dehydrated level of 3% will still take several hours to reach full hydration even with regular drinks. For those in a warm climate where sweating continues during re-hydration it will take longer, and for severe de-hydration in any climate full recovery can take over 24 hours. In severe cases it's important to include electrolytes with water otherwise the balance in body salts and particularly a severe reduction in sodium levels can be dangerous.

3.4 Hydration and Creatine supplementation.

Many athletes, powerlifters and weight trainees take creatine monohydrate or similar creatine compounds as a supplement. This is entirely WADA legal as well as being sensible, why? It's a natural part of meat and fish and all the reliable medical studies prove supplementation is effective at improving both strength and power as well as reducing recovery time. This is particularly true for those athletes who eat little or no meat as they have to synthesise it from a mixture of amino acids from a limited vegetable diet which reduces the amount of protein amino acids for muscle recovery. Creatine requires additional water intake for storage in the muscles otherwise it may create a false dehydration. Imagine the muscles acting like a sponge trying to absorb water from the rest of the body and this will give you an idea of the affect. Without additional fluid intake the supplement may cause severe dehydration which can lead to cramping as well as reducing the positive effect of the creatine on strength due to the negative effect of the dehydration. If in doubt, follow the instructions on the creatine package and increase your fluid intake as suggested. The urine colour test should be used regularly when supplementing with creatine to ensure the benefits are seen. When you stop supplementing it's important to maintain this additional fluid intake for up to four weeks as the additional muscle stores will remain elevated for some time.

3.5 Muscle stores of Creatine phosphate

Creatine, as the compound phosphocreatine (PCr) plays a key role in the chemical reactions of ATP and the subsequent release of energy in muscle contraction. The chemical pathways to re-generate ATP and maintain muscle contractions is complex and a high level of creatine phosphate resident as a reservoir in the muscles makes a significant difference to the power and duration of a muscle's capability. The usual supplement is creatine monohydrate, although other compounds are available. Supplementation has been shown to significantly reduce the time for recovery of muscle creatine phosphate stores and also to reduce the level of muscle soreness following exercise. Because of this, it's an important issue in the recovery from training to normalisation. Without supplementation the creatine storage levels return to near normal in 24-48 hours post exercise and may remain a little elevated for some time depending on the condition of the individual, diet and the intensity of the muscular stress. Supplementation has been extensively studied and the general consensus is that it influences the recovery timeline in several ways:

1.   Faster ATP re-synthesis.
2.   Faster muscle glycogen storage replacement.
3.   Reduced muscle damage from training and reduced inflammation.
4.   Improved muscle fibre protein synthesis during the adaptation supper compensation stage.

Creatine in the muscles immediately starts to recover after exercise and goes on to super compensate a little if the available amino acids or ingested creatine is available. The elevated levels from a single session can last for up to several days depending on the intensity of the exercise and the availability before returning to normal base levels if no further exercise is undertaken. With regular exercise the levels remain higher than those of sedentary individuals even without supplementation, assuming diet is adequate. While the advantages of taking creatine as a supplement are well understood, the actual improvement in recovery time has not been demonstrated specifically other than to suggest a range of between 10-30% improvement compared to similar individuals who are not taking creatine supplements. This faster recovery between exercise sets and post exercise is an important factor in the recovery process and must be considered an advantage.

3.6 ATP/ATD.

Now, this is where the rubber hits the road. At the very heart of energy production in a muscle ATP produces the energy for the protein links to contract. Our muscles contain a small amount of this ATP chemical, but it reacts when required with other chemicals, notably creatine phosphate to provide a free phosphate energy molecule that is used to contract protein links when triggered by the signal from the brain. When ATP loses its phosphate molecule it becomes ATD which is then converted back to ATP via several complex processes depending on the intensity of the muscle action, to be ready for further action in this cyclic process. The cycle of ATP/ATD uses different fuels appropriate for the immediacy and intensity of the muscle action required and also produces different waste products depending on the re-generation mode in operation. In reality several of the modes may be active at any one time to a greater or lesser extent. Each mode has a different efficiency and speed for producing and cycling ATD to ATP ranging from very fast for immediate high intensity muscle contractions using creatine phosphate to a slower and steady production for extreme endurance activity using fats and glycogen. The biological processes for these actions are very complex. If you want chapter and verse I suggest you look on the internet for the schematic diagrams and chemical reactions. However, here are the primary modes of ATP/ADP production during exercise listed in order of speed, or 'selection' by the CNS when we exercise. Below they are described very briefly.

1. Phosphocreatine (PCr System (Anaerobic Alactic System):
PCr is stored in muscles and can rapidly donate a phosphate group to ADP to regenerate ATP. This system is highly efficient, but limited in duration, typically providing energy for high-intensity activities lasting up to 10-15 seconds.

2. Glycolytic System (Anaerobic Lactic System):
Glycolysis is the breakdown of glucose (glycogen) to produce ATP. This process occurs in the cytoplasm and doesn't require oxygen. It provides energy for high-intensity activities lasting from 30 seconds to about 2 minutes. The end product of glycolysis pyruvate, can be converted to lactate when oxygen is limited. Accumulation of lactate will lead to muscle fatigue.

3. Oxidative System (Aerobic System):
Aerobic metabolism occurs in the mitochondria and relies on the presence of oxygen. It utilizes carbohydrates, fats, and to a lesser extent proteins to produce ATP through the Krebs cycle (citric acid cycle) and oxidative phosphorylation. This system provides energy for longer-duration, lower-intensity activities, such as endurance exercises like long-distance running or cycling.

4. Beta-Oxidation:
This is a metabolic pathway that breaks down fatty acids to produce acetyl-CoA, which enters the Krebs cycle to generate ATP. Beta-oxidation primarily fuels endurance activities when carbohydrate stores become depleted.

5. Protein Catabolism:
Under extreme conditions or very prolonged exercise, proteins can be broken down into amino acids and converted to glucose (gluconeogenesis) or directly enter the Krebs cycle to produce ATP. This should be avoided at all costs by the strength athlete, so multi-marathon running is not an option if you want to gain strength!

As you will no doubt realise these processes are very complex and only briefly detailed here. With respect to recovery, ATP is re-generated during exercise and will continue to do so post exercise to reach normal levels during which time you will use more oxygen and usually glycogen than at normal resting rates to fuel the process. Consequently, having appropriate carbohydrate intake after exercise is important for rapid ATP recovery. Most individuals will recover quickly within hours, although following extremely intense exercise such as long distance running this may extend to 24 hours. From my research I can find no mention of ATP overcompensating in any way or taking longer than 24 hours to recover even in extreme cases provided adequate fuels are available. Having a good store of creatine in the muscles helps fast recovery using the phosphocreatine system following short bursts of intense muscular contraction, because of this effect creatine supplementation is a no brain choice for any athlete.

3.7 Glycogen.

Glycogen is the primary fuel for both fast twitch muscular contraction (the strong ones) and initially the slower contraction motor units (the endurance ones), it's severely depleted with high levels of intense muscular activity of any duration. Levels recover quickly if the blood and gut contain adequate sugars and carbohydrates. Glycogen storage super compensates within 2-3 days following an intense training event assuming adequate carbohydrate ingestion and rest, this lasts for a further 2-5 days. This over compensation is of lower importance to the pure strength athlete training anaerobic muscular functions for short bursts of intense activity. However, it's important for those with both strength and endurance elements in their training or sport, e.g. rugby. In general, glycogen is the primary source of fuel for most sports except for long distance low intensity activity where triglyceride (fat) becomes the main source of energy as the stored glycogen in the body becomes depleted. The overcompensation following an intense draining of glycogen can be used to artificially raise glycogen storage levels with a process known as carbohydrate loading. Loading is a nutritional strategy that can be used by athletes to maximise muscle glycogen stores before an endurance event, competition or planned prolonged exercise. The goal of carbohydrate loading is to enhance performance by providing the muscles with a greater readily available source of energy. Here's how carbohydrate loading typically works:

Depletion Phase:
Athletes first engage in a period of glycogen depletion through intense training combined with a low-carbohydrate diet. The purpose of this phase is to reduce muscle glycogen stores, making the muscles more responsive to carbohydrate intake during the subsequent loading phase. The time taken is usually 3-7 days.

Loading Phase:
After the depletion phase, athletes switch to a high-carbohydrate diet while reducing training intensity. This phase usually lasts 1-3 days and involves consuming large amounts of carbohydrates often accounting for 70-80% of total daily caloric intake. The increased carbohydrate intake maximises muscle glycogen stores beyond normal levels.
The science behind carbohydrate loading revolves around the body's response to glycogen depletion and the subsequent super compensation of glycogen stores. When muscle glycogen stores are depleted through intense exercise and a low-carbohydrate diet the muscles become more sensitive to insulin, which drives a greater amount into storage when loading.

Carbohydrates also influence the production of neurotransmitters like serotonin, which plays a role in mood regulation and emotional well-being. Adequate carbohydrate intake helps to stabilise mood and reduce feelings of fatigue or irritability, thereby supporting overall mental capacity and productivity. For those of you who know body builders, you will understand how irritable they become on a low carb diet. Carbohydrate loading is most beneficial for endurance athletes participating in events lasting longer than 90 minutes, such as marathons, triathlons, cycling races, and long-distance swimming. Carbohydrate loading should only be used infrequently and if the individual is in perfect health.

3.8 Fat.
Triglyceride, the fat stored within, and around muscles, and in many places in the body is used as fuel for slow twitch muscle activity such as distance running and endurance sports. This does not appear to have any recovery requirements or super compensate in any manner. During long duration activity, fat is mobilised from stores throughout the body by the secretion of enzymes in the liver, releasing fat into the blood for immediate use as fuel. Fat cells will replenish if calorie intake exceeds energy requirements for normal activity, but without an excess calorie intake the fat storage cannot re-fill, this is observed in typical lean body types of long distance runners and bodybuilders who expend far more energy than consumed when 'cutting' for a competition. There is some evidence that previously laid down fat cells are more easily refilled than the deposit of new ones, however this is not super compensation. Low repetition heavy strength exercise does not use triglyceride as fuel, for this reason fat is only an issue for strength athletes having to remain in a competition weight category, and for aesthetic reasons.

3.9 CNS Recovery.
The brain and CNS recovery is often overlooked. Recent research into this subject suggests that the brain and associated nervous system may take 48 hours or longer to recover lost hormones and chemicals such as creatine and serotonin after violent or highly stressful muscle contractions. Practical experience supports this as a disinclination to train hard again after an intense session. The possible super compensation of the chemicals used in driving muscular contractions in the brain has yet to be examined robustly, despite this we may assume there are some changes following severe muscular stress leading to improved capability after a recovery period.

3.10 Vascular development.
Growth in vascular capillaries and fluid storage is stimulated by a high volume of exercise repetition and less so with low numbers of heavy repetitions. Improved vascular capacity and swollen muscles is a popular bodybuilders aim. The increased blood flow can last for several hours, and when continually repeated in workout sessions may last partially for several days. This is known as the bodybuilders 'pump' where the muscle becomes swollen with additional fluid and blood. It may look impressive, but does not improve strength. Regular training, using higher repetitions increases the fluid retention in the muscle's surrounding tissues, which becomes semi permanent with ongoing training. Such training is thought to allow marginally faster recovery from exercise due to the improved blood flow to the area, but this is anecdotal. Consequently, it's not considered as an issue in recovery.

3.11 Delayed onset muscle soreness (DOMS).

The obvious sign that unusual or excessive muscle stress has occurred is the soreness and stiffness known as 'delayed onset muscle soreness' (DOMS) which occurs 12-48 hours after a hard workout. It may last for up to 5 days in severe cases. Beginners to weight training often suffer from this after relatively light workouts where the same exercises and weights used would have no consequence whatsoever for a stronger athlete, or that same individual a year later into their training plans. Whether DOMS is present or not after training, the damaged muscle protein links must be cleared and replaced. Two simultaneous processes deal with this every day whether you train or not, they are; catabolism, (removal) and anabolism (replacement). Every day your muscles undergo minor renewal, but after unusual stress, such as heavy weight training the inflammation from damage and the following repair is hugely increased. This muscle fibre damage and swelling can be very uncomfortable, and in some cases debilitating. You could think of it like a brick building that has undergone a sudden shock, broken bricks need to be removed and replaced with new ones cemented in place to repair the structure. Then, the following super compensation may be likened to the builder adding an extra layer of bricks to protect the building from similar shocks in the future.

Many trainees seek this DOMS as a badge of honour, demonstrating that they are working the muscles hard, and they are right, but at what expense? Having DOMS inevitably means your recovery time must be extended and in some cases the damage will restrict super compensation in favour of injury repair.

3.12 Hypertrophy.

Last, but by no means least we come to the structural recovery of muscles and supportive tissues. While all the other issues mentioned above are resolving, the minor structural damage to the muscles is cleared and repaired prior to structural additions, namely hypertrophy.

This complex process driven by hormonal signals from the damaged tissues and the CNS starts with catabolism clearing damaged tissue, and anabolism replacing it with new and additional protein links if the amino acids are available. This process usually takes between 3-10 days where the nutrients are freely available, depending on the level of micro damage and the individual's health and activity during the recovery period. Anabolism is highly dependent on various hormones, notably testosterone and takes far longer for individuals with low levels of this important hormone. Testosterone levels start falling significantly for men over the age of 40 and the decline is reflected in extended recovery time.

Medical evidence shows that continued heavy resistance training maintains a high level of testosterone into later years. While hypertrophy is the goal of many, it's a sad fact that 90% or more of the individuals I see in gyms never allow this process to complete before repeating their training, hence the attraction of steroids that accelerate anabolism artificially with all the unpleasant side effects.

4. LOCAL AND SYSTEMIC RECOVERY.

Localised recovery takes a relatively short time with most of the issues listed in the previous chapter returning to normal within 24 hours, if the health, diet and lifestyle of the individual is supportive. However, even the most basic requirement of oxygen needs the support of the whole body to achieve. Consequently there is a systemic, or whole body recovery process encompassing the minor local deficits and waste product removal alongside the protracted muscle repair processes. The greater the exercise debt built from a workout, the greater the recovery period, and training again before recovery is pointless and even counter productive. This debt is built from a combination of intensity and duration of exercise as well as the size of the muscles used. Clearly a smaller muscles like the biceps will incur less debt that a larger muscle such as the quadriceps if both are exercised to a similar level of stress. Mike Mentzer, one of the most famous bodybuilders in the 1970's and a great thinker was vociferous on the subject of recovery and he wrote many articles and several books on the subject of building strength and muscle size where he promoted the high intensity low duration approach to training. His ideas were often ridiculed and dismissed by the contemporary mainstream despite good medical evidence supporting his views. It was mainly his methods that took me from a puny 10 stone to 15 stone and four national powerlifting titles. Yes, it did! His methods were much later adopted in part by top bodybuilders and strength athletes including the multi-Olympia winner Dorian Yates. The essence of his approach consisted of very short, low set, high intensity training to muscle failure and beyond using rest pause, static and eccentric contractions after normal concentric failure. This was followed by far longer rest periods between workouts than used by just about every other elite bodybuilder at that time. He typically advised only 1 or 2 sets for each body part using a 3 or 4 way split, resting between 4 and 7 days between each workout. To clarify this, for a 3 way body split this would mean between 12 and 21 days in the cycle to cover all muscle groups. The contemporary plans using 5 or 6 training days a week in common use was advised against, and he suggested that such plans would never allow full recovery between sessions if true high intensity to complete muscle failure was performed in each exercise. He argued that once a muscle had been taken to extreme failure the conditions for growth had been stimulated and there was no point in performing further sets as this would only increase muscle damage, systemic debt within the body and extend the time to recovery and super-compensation. Some of his plans advised only 1 working set after a short warm up for each body part. It should be remembered, that in the 19070's steroids to enhance muscle growth became available driving anabolism and reducing recovery times to the point where bodybuilders could train virtually every day and still make gains. This steroid abuse has led to the predominant approach over the last 40 years where multiple exercises and high sets for each body part are used which indulges the genetically gifted and drug using bodybuilder. In fact, it's an unfortunate truth that now, to be an elite bodybuilder you have to join the drug train. The high set, high repetition methods are so entrenched that even beginners assume that's the only way to build muscle, they misunderstand in their enthusiasm and haste that those promoting such plans are drug users. Consequently, after struggling to make any substantial gains using these deceptive training plans they often join the drug train. The methods Mentzer proposed rely on far longer rest periods to allow recovery and adaptation of the muscles and are proven by medical science as ideal for a clean athlete, be it for strength or bodybuilding.

We know from medical evidence that whenever we put great stress on our body through intense exercise the whole body has to contribute to the recovery. For example, a long distance runner will use the leg muscle creatine and glycogen reserves initially, and then the whole body contributes to the sustained effort through providing these compounds and triglyceride into the blood supply.

Similarly, when you stress an individual muscle group with intense weight training the whole body contributes both locally and systemically to sustain the action and the following recovery. Clearly localised resources are used up first.   After a leg workout they will feel weakened, but you wouldn't expect your arms to ache or feel weak. The whole body contributes systemically to enable recovery and an intense leg workout depletes the body's overall capacity to recover. This makes an arm workout less productive when undertaken shortly after an intense leg session. Hence Mike Mentzer's recommendation to only train every 4-7 days.

Your CNS also has to recover from highly intense exercise and your brain will constrain your resolve to continue or repeat the same any time soon. If you already train with weights you will recognise this subtle sapping of the will. For example, you may plan to complete six sets of squats with a weight you can manage for 6 repetitions, but after the second set you may start to think 'that's enough, I'll do more next week'. The CNS systemic debt is building and your brain wants to conserve energy to recover, its avoidance of systemic debt is a built in survival mechanism, so maintaining motivation in such situations requires consistent ongoing training and mental strength.

Recovery towards the super compensation phase may be considered as two separate parallel processes as shown in **Fig.8** as local and systemic. The local recovery begins very quickly the

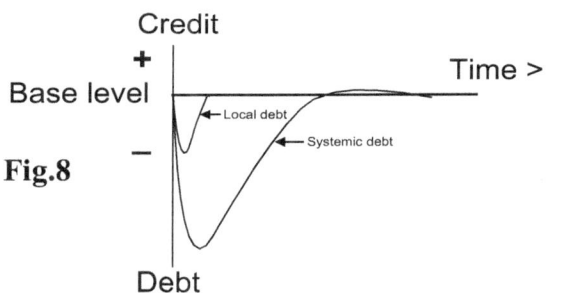

Fig.8

moment you stop exercising with creatine, ATP and other muscle chemicals building within minutes while any lactic acid build up starts clearing. That's why you can perform one weight training exercise set to failure, and then another in only a couple of minutes. While local recovery may be quick, systemic debt builds with the volume of intense exercise and can take a very long time to resolve. Because of this, after achieving the desired stress stimulus on a muscle to kick start adaptation it's undesirable to continue with further unnecessary stress. More sets and repetitions will simply add to the systemic debt and lengthen the recovery time without adding any increase in super compensation. Following any intense muscular action the local depletion and some systemic debt must be partially repaid before exercise on another body part can be fully productive. After 5 sets of 3 repetitions squatting to true failure, it's just not productive to do the same with the deadlift anytime soon. If you do you're kidding yourself it's anywhere near your best. The quadriceps and the posterior chain will be severely depleted and the CNS is exhausted from the effort. You will have dug a deep hole in your reserves. The locally used muscles will recover a high percentage of their function and capacity in several hours, but repeating anything like it with the same intensity is impossible for days, and in some cases weeks. Yes, you read that correctly, for some individuals it has been shown that full recovery may take weeks, and in fact may never super compensate if the stress is excessive. Damage to the protein links within individual fibres must be repaired and the muscles returned slowly to normal, then beyond into super compensation. Systemic debt can't be recovered without adequate time passing as organic compounds have to be replaced. These come through diet and digestion, the action of the liver and kidneys, and from catabolism and anabolism within the body itself. This all takes time to complete, we are not machines and the body cannot be rushed without

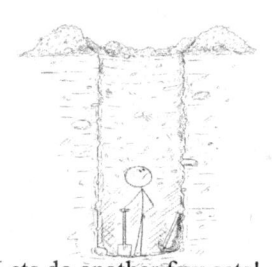

Lets do another few sets!

artificial hormones. Several muscle functions rebound from intense exercise stress into over compensating as a body defence mechanism as explained in the previous chapters. Muscle growth and strength increases from CNS adaptation are only triggered by 'unusual' muscular stress and the individual muscle fibres hypertrophy through added contractile proteins and improved vascular capacity. The trigger levels that cause this compensation to occur cannot be numerically defined as they are different for each individual and for the same individual at different times in their development. What we do know is that once spent, the debt has to be repaid, and just like your credit card, paying it off becomes difficult if you spend too much. Don't dig yourself into a big black hole!

5. THE INDIVIDUALAITY OF RECOVERY

Recovery to a point where you're into super compensation and ready to train again to build upon the additional strength and growth is highly individual. There are guidelines from medical and practical experience, but the numerous factors involved make accuracy difficult. The chart in **Fig.9**

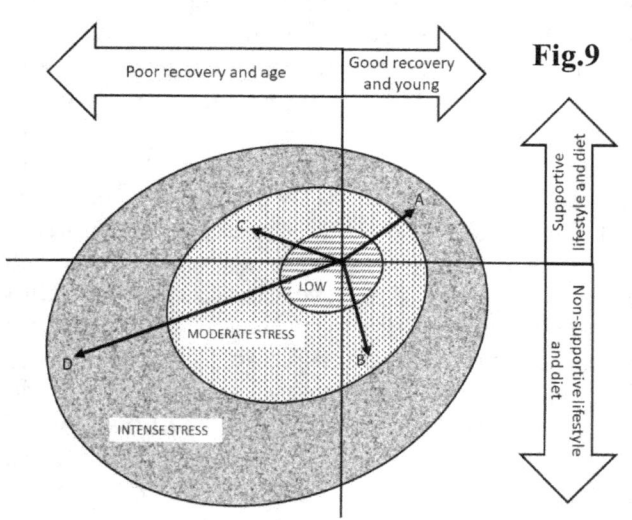

Fig.9

is not to scale, but represents some of this individuality. Above the centre line and to the right represents individuals who are both young and have a supportive lifestyle and diet. As you can see the return path to the centre representing full recovery is far shorter from any stress level in this quadrant. Those in this section will recover quickly from all training including high intensity. On the other hand individuals below the centre line and towards the left will experience longer delays to recovery from at all but the lowest intensity levels. The bands of low, moderate and high intensity represent the range of variable intensity of stress. This intensity is also subject to the individuals 'perception' of how hard they train. For many individuals I have observed and coached their perception of what is intense training is often very short of reality. Lets look at a simple example using **Fig.9**. Four gym friends decide to train legs together. Alan is 18, (A) he pushes himself very hard to complete muscle failure on most sets and for him the intensity is both perceived and actually high. Alan also has a very supportive lifestyle with an excellent high protein diet, he uses good recovery protocols such as constant hydration, regular creatine supplementation and he enjoys low stress work and excellent sleep. He returns to full recovery represented by the centre point on the chart in around 5-6 days. Brian (B) is the same age as Alan, but he eases through the workout without putting everything into it. He grunted a bit and thought he was training hard, but his effort was well short of actual muscle failure. As a consequence, his intensity could only be considered as moderately high as shown by point B.

Brian like his booze and has a chaotic lifestyle with a poor diet resulting in his recovery line to the centre point being around 6-7 days despite the intensity being in the moderate range. Colin (C) is in his 40's and like Brian eases through the workout stopping well short of being 'all in' resulting in his intensity being moderate at point C. He has a reasonably supportive lifestyle with an acceptable diet and a low stress job, so due to this he is likely to recover to the centre point in 5 -6 days. David (D) is in his 50's and pushes himself very hard like Alan in the workout perceiving it correctly as very intense, resulting in his intensity at point D. However, David does not eat well at all and his job places him under a lot of daily stress. With late nights, poor sleep and numerous worries his poor lifestyle results in his recovery to the centre point being in excess of 13 days.

The point I am making here is that you can never be entirely precise about recovery times. Our lives are never constant and stress levels from work and relationships along with varying diet and other physical work done in the meantime impacts directly on recovery. In the situation above, if all else remains constant and the group train weekly, Alan will make good progress. Brian and Colin, due to a lack of intensity will make slow progress. David is unlikely to make any progress and is actually at risk of injury from doing the same workout a week later while still deep into early recovery. As you should now appreciate, recovery is not an exact science and will vary considerably between individuals who are apparently doing the same workout.

When I talk to people in the gyms I use, I am often asked how I manage to lift so much weight and maintain my muscle mass in my 70's. I advise low set low reps and training to failure with lots of rest between sessions, good nutrition and a simple split doing no more than 3 sessions a week giving each muscle group at least 7 days rest. How simple is that? But alas, when I watch from across the gym I see how they ignore my advice and train like maniacs. They get nowhere, digging a deeper and deeper recovery hole before in frustration they join the train. Ho Hum.

Remember, if you're healthy and training, but not gaining strength and muscle size there can only be a few simple reasons for a lack of progress:

1.   You're not training intensely enough to stimulate your CNS and growth.
2.   You're not recovering from your training between working the same muscles.
3.   You're not fuelling your body correctly.
4.   You have reached your full genetic potential.

Number 4 is very, very unlikely.

6. MUSCLE PROTEIN CATABOLISM AND ANABOLISM

The catabolic process of clearing the debris from damaged muscle protein links, and the anabolic reconstruction is the longest of the recovery processes. It may be uneventful and without any apparent discomfort when the damage is low. However, where DOMS is experienced the duration of recovery will inevitably be longer. Heavy eccentric training in particular ('negatives' where the muscle lengthens under heavy load) generates severe DOMS as it causes an abnormal level of micro trauma in the muscles. Recovery takes time, energy, and the function of key internal organs to achieve, so body size, age, illness and personal abuse with drugs or alcohol will extend the recovery time for any individual. The affect of varying levels of exercise intensity on human muscle is well understood from many scientific studies. We know that very low levels of stress, or no activity will result in the body removing muscle tissue via atrophy. Muscle wastage occurs naturally where a muscle is under used, for example a leg in plaster from a broken bone or a lazy person not wanting to walk anywhere. Unlike fat, muscle needs a constant blood supply to provide nutrients and energy to maintain its existing size. The body has to use precious resource daily to maintain muscle tissue and we have evolved with body functions to conserve energy for survival. Consequently, excessive muscle tissue is unwanted as far as your body is concerned. Your body would eagerly eat itself given the opportunity, and underused muscle will be reduced in size by catabolism as an entirely normal consequence of its lack of use. My father was a big man, he had strong muscular legs, but in his 80's through illness he didn't walk far and his legs turned to matchsticks. The phrase 'use it or lose it' applies very well to human muscle. To maintain existing

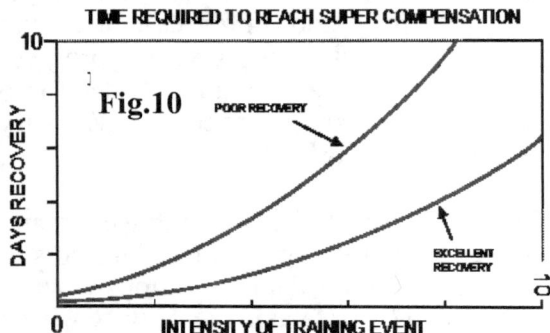

muscle it must be mildly stressed on a regular basis to ensure the CNS considers it as necessary and required for the future. The relationship between the intensity of muscle contraction and atrophy, maintenance or hypertrophy is highly individual and relevant to current conditioning. This also applies to recovery and varies as we have already discussed. Recovery may be poor or excellent and everything in between as represented in **Fig.10**. Note that in the extreme stress range the recovery from high stress goes off the scale for some individuals. The return to homeostasis and beyond into super compensation has been extensively studied by medical science with many results well documented and **Fig.11** shows a typical result that's been repeated in experiments in universities around the world. This particular graph shows

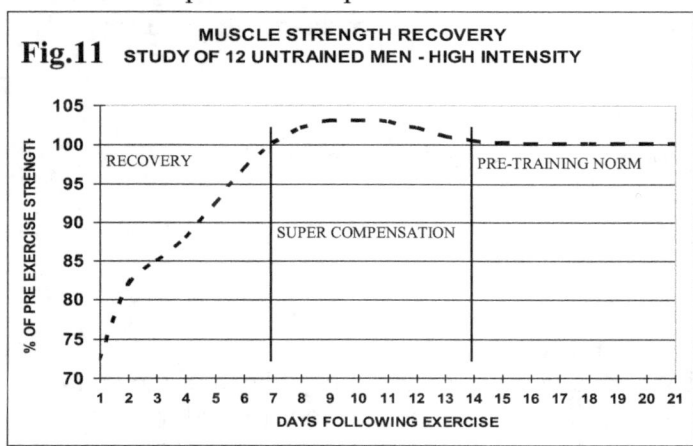

the recovery time measured as pure strength where 12 untrained healthy young men were put onto a high intensity, low volume quadriceps training plan using a leg extension machine. The study was followed by monitoring of blood waste products and muscle amino acid synthesis, as well as regular muscle strength tests. The results showed that <u>on average</u> the base level of strength was regained in 7 days, followed by 7 days of super compensation tapering to normal pre-training event levels. The advantage of the super compensation phase could be accrued with additional training within days 8-14 following the initial training event. But, take careful note, these were fit young men and on day 7 they had only just reached 100% of their previous strength without any further other high stress on other body parts. Are you training legs hard once or even more every week and doing lots of other stuff as well and wondering why gains are so slow or have stopped altogether? **<u>Now you may have an idea why!</u>**

The full potential from super compensation was found to be between 9 and 11 days, again note that no other exercise was involved. These figures are the average from the medically controlled experiment and some individuals took far longer while others took a little less time to reach super compensation. I used to coach one guy who holds the British bench press record, the 2009/10 European title, IPF World championship silver medallist, and is the British GBPF record holder in two body weights. He trained every week with an intensity that would kill me yet recovered fully in 4-6 days. He was able to continue this sequence using a step training pattern (one day heavy, one day light technique) for the bench press twice a week virtually indefinitely. However, and this is the important point, he only trained for the bench press and rarely trained legs or back. At one time he decided to start training for the squat and deadlift as well, intending to compete in three lift competitions. He did this all within the weekly microcycle and his bench performance dropped off alarmingly. The weights he would normally double could not be lifted for singles. We discussed what he had been doing, stopped the leg and back work and within two weeks his bench press was back on track. It was clear to me that his greater systemic debt from the leg and back work extended his recovery from the bench sessions. Even the strongest people in the world are subject to normal biology, so if you think you're different, think again!

From the medical study results above, you will now understand that a beginners training programme where each muscle group is trained two or even three times a week can only be a preparation phase. During this time the exercises stimulate the CNS to learn synchronous and movement coordination. Beyond the beginners phase your whole body can't continue training with maximum intensity or anywhere near it three times a week. If you tried, after 3 weeks you'd be a wreck or by default a chemical cheat. If you think you can get your full strength back in 3-4 days after a hard leg workout and you're not on steroids, then you're either a different species to the rest of us or more likely your training falls well short of highly intense. Which do you think is more likely? This raises several important issues for your own programme, or those you provide for others:

1. The study results shown here are repeatable anywhere in the world with similar results. This particular study (**Fig.11**) used 12 young healthy men. If you fall outside this category recovery is likely to take longer. As you age, or if you're living an unhealthy lifestyle the metabolic processes and capacity of key organs are reduced and recovery time will increase. Older men in particular start to lose their testosterone level which also extends recovery. Make an honest assessment of your lifestyle and health. Are you at the bottom, or the top of the recovery band?

2. The impact of more workouts following the initial training event and the cumulative systemic and localised effect on recovery isn't included in **Fig.11.** Any repeated systemic depletion from intense sessions such as separate squats, deadlifts and other exercises or sports are not factored into the graph above. You can't isolate a workout with regards to systemic body functions. While you may recover in 7 days from a hard leg session in isolation, you will probably do chest, back and arms before training legs again. These muscles will also require recovery, both local and systemic, which will extend the super compensation for your legs out to 8-10 days or beyond. If you train several times a week, even on different body parts with honest intensity, then a weekly, seven day plan may need extending to 10 days or more. Oh dear!

3. Well trained strength athletes have a faster metabolism and acclimatisation to muscle stress and can generally recover quicker. This is accelerated by steroid usage, allowing more training in less time. None of the data here considers this drug abuse, if you want details on training with steroids give this booklet away and look elsewhere for books on how to cheat, there are plenty of them about.

If you're healthy and have a good recovery capacity, you should avoid training any major muscle group <u>intensely</u> more than once every 7 days and preferably every 8 or 9. For those over 40 years of age or with a less than perfect lifestyle and health, I suggest a long period of several months low intensity work preparing the body before attempting high intensity training, otherwise you will simply burn out. As you get stronger and bigger you will need to schedule more recovery time, or add recovery protocols such as massage and full days of rest. Good nutrition helps considerably, particularly appropriate and timely protein intake immediately following a workout.

7. TESTING YOUR RECOVERY

Without complicated equipment, heart rate monitors, blood sampling and a whole load of medical staff you're unable to determine accurately your recovery time for any muscle group. However, predicting it through trial and error is easy for any individual muscle using an isolation exercise, or a general muscle group with a compound exercise. Testing the largest muscle groups using a compound exercise will give you your longest recovery period to start with. The major muscle groups in your legs take the longest time to reach super compensation because they have the largest muscle mass in your body, and larger muscles take longer to recover from intense stress. When you next train your legs, choose one compound exercise such as the squat, deadlift or leg press and include 3 sets of 6 repetitions in the plan for that exercise. It's important to choose a test exercise you're already performing regularly otherwise the CNS, which needs to learn better coordination for any new exercise will quickly adapt and skew the result. Choose a weight that's difficult for you to complete 6 repetitions with. Take a full 5 minutes between the sets and perform all three with the same weight to complete muscle failure without any spotters aiding you to complete repetitions. Add up the total number of repetitions achieved for the three sets. When you're due to work your legs again, repeat this test with the same weight at the same point in your workout. Remember to avoid any duplication of training on that muscle or group before testing again. If you can perform more repetitions in total, then you've recovered fully and are in the super compensation phase. If not, then count the repetitions achieved and repeat the process, adding two days to your rest period before attempting the test again. Repeat this process if the total repetitions achieved is the same or lower than previously until you find the right recovery period. **Fig.12** shows an example of how this may look when completed. The leg press exercise may take 9 days to show an improvement, while smaller muscles such as calves may show improvement in 5 days. Some individuals find it shocking when they discover that they need 10 days or more to see an increase in repetitions for the larger muscles. With this knowledge, you can start to plan the post training rest periods correctly to drive real progress. Now, this can lead to a training plan with variable rest periods between different exercises. For example, some powerlifters who understand their own recovery capability only train the deadlift for 1RM every 14 or 21 days, alternating the squat and deadlift weekly while training the bench press twice or more in the same period. For those that feel the need to train all three power lifts weekly, doing

RECOVERY TEST					
Fig.12	3X6 TOTAL REPETITIONS				
TEST EXERCISE	WEIGHT	REPS	TEST 1-DAY +5	TEST 2-DAY +7	TEST 3-DAY +9
LEG PRESS	250	19	17	19	21
BICEP CURL	40	18	19		
PEC DECK	55	17	16	18	
CALF RAISE	35	20	21		

this without becoming over trained will need a wave or step training system. For example, with 'load' (maximum weights) alternating with 'deload' (50% max) and 'reload' (75% max) over a 14 or 21 day cycle. An example is shown in **Fig.13.** You will note that none of the three powerlifting exercises are trained to 1RM levels in the same week. These training methods are explained in detail in 'The Strength Coach Training Techniques and Methods', or 'Coaching Powerlifters'. Remember, if you're not progressing, barring injury, illness or lowering testosterone levels, it can only be due to a very limited number of reasons. They are; a lack of applied training intensity,

Example rotational 3 phase plan			Fig.13
21 DAY CYCLE	SQUAT	DEADLIFT	BENCH
WEEK 1	1RM	50% 1RM	50% 1RM
WEEK 2	50% 1RM	1RM	75% 1RM
WEEK 3	75% 1RM	75% 1RM	1RM

inadequate recovery time, or diet and lifestyle problems, it's not rocket science!

8. RECOVERY AIDS AND BLOCKERS

There are several actions you can take that will help your recovery, and conversely some that slow or stop it completely. Here's a list of the more important issues:

AIDS
1. **GOOD HYDRATION.** Fluid replacement is essential for the efficient removal of waste products and the storage of muscle glycogen and phosphor creatine for the muscle contraction process. Good hydration must be a high priority during, and immediately after intense exercise. Getting cramps in the evening, or the night after a workout is a clear indicator that you're dehydrated. Muscle strength will diminish very quickly with dehydration; a 2% reduction in body weight from dehydration has been shown to reduce 1RM by up to 10%, so for the strength athlete or sportsman this is a critical issue, you need to get it right.
2. **EAT CARBOHYDRATES.** Severe diets restrict glycogen storage recovery and super compensation within the muscles. You require carbohydrates for easy conversion to blood sugar and hence the replacement of glycogen in the muscle stores. Without a good supply of carbohydrates immediately post workout your body is unable to compensate directly from blood sugar and catabolism may have to convert stored fat or even muscle protein to glycogen. While this is good for fat loss, it will delay your recovery and will reduce the possible glycogen over compensation.

3. EAT MORE PROTEIN. It's proven that your exercised muscles are more receptive to new protein synthesis within the first 3 hours after intense strength exercise. Following this, protein synthesis returns to normal. To take advantage of this window of opportunity you need free amino acids in your blood as soon as possible after training. Supplementation immediately before, or after a workout with an appropriate fast absorption protein source is an excellent method. Low protein diets will delay or minimise any super compensation and may result in the catabolism of existing muscle tissue elsewhere in the body to replace protein degraded in the muscles stressed.

4. EAT REGULARLY. We know the timely supply of basic nutrients will aid recovery, and the maintenance of these in the blood supply at optimum levels will ensure recovery is maximised. Regular small meals (up to six a day) containing carbohydrate, protein and natural balanced ingredients that contain essential vitamins are best. However, with busy lives this isn't always possible. Use supplements if appropriate meals are not easily available to optimise recovery over the days following a workout, but be careful not to exceed your daily calorie intake with some supplements, otherwise you will just get fat.

5. CREATINE MONOHYDRATE. Intense exercise depletes the creatine phosphate stored within the muscles that must be replaced from diet directly, or synthesised by the liver from ingested amino acids. The levels stored within the muscles may be elevated considerably from normal via a 'loading up' process. Loading is achieved over 5 days with high doses of 20 grams a day or over longer periods with smaller doses. Loading is proven to have a positive result on muscle strength during intense exercise and in recovery, once loaded a 3-5 gram dose a day will maintain the loaded state.

6. GET QUALITY REST AND SLEEP. Put your feet up, read a book, watch a film, have a long lie in. While resting you're not using much energy and your body recovers quicker. Sleep is a vital part of recovery and you should aim for 8 hours every night. Some medical evidence suggests muscle growth is more likely during sleep so this is a serious issue for the strength athlete. If something is disturbing your sleep then resolve it quickly.

7. STRETCH AND MASSAGE. Stretch and massage the areas being exercised or preferably get someone else to do it. This stimulates the blood supply to the area and increases the supply of nutrients to the muscles. Results are anecdotal from massage, but it certainly won't extend recovery. Vibration devices may help recovery by doing the same thing. Several recent studies have proven that these vibration devices used before and again after intense strength exercise helps recovery by stimulating the blood supply to the area. It's also good practice to massage muscles and joints where the tendons attach to bones during a workout between sets, this increases blood flow and warms the area to help prevent injuries.

8. LIGHT RECOVERY EXERCISE. Some sports therapists recommend very light training of the exercised muscles the following day to increase blood supply and possibly reduce the duration of DOMS. Typically, around 50 light repetitions of the same exercise the next day, but don't overdo it, excessive cardio work extends recovery and could stop it altogether. Keep it light, repeating intense exercise simply drives the body into chronic fatigue, avoid it!

9. WATER MASSAGE/HOT TUBS. One study showed that 20 minutes of underwater jet massage therapy 3 times per week might help maintain performance capacity during intense training. The results are generally anecdotal rather than proven, but it can't hurt, so if you've access to such facilities use them.

10. **HOT AND COLD.** This is often used by sports therapists to reduce swelling and DOMS. Alternate cold ice packs with warm covers while stretching and massaging the exercises area. You may get a similar effect from alternating a sauna with a cold shower.

11. **COLD BATHS.** Again, often used by sports therapists, but very uncomfortable and unproven as an aid to recovery by medical science. Some sports therapists advise sitting in a cold water bath for 15 minutes after a very intense session. A short swim in cold water is less traumatic if you have the facilities nearby.

12. **MUSCLE COMPRESSION.** Often used as part of a sport therapist routine. Elastic bandages or sleeves that can be applied to the arms and legs are readily available. The consequence on recovery is anecdotal and unproven, but it's likely to reduce any swelling and may improve recovery. It's worth using, particularly on any problem area or old injury site such as a knee or elbow.

13. **ELECTRICAL MUSCLE STIMULATION.** Many of these machines are advertised as toners or even muscle trainers. The claims for fitness and muscular toning made by some manufacturers are very suspect with some claims clearly outrageous. One advert shows before, and after results with totally ripped abdominals from using a toner, bloody ridiculous! Having said this, they may be useful in remedial situations to help an injury recover. Some reliable reports suggest light contractions using one of these devices on a stressed muscle will have the same impact as light exercise or massage and may reduce recovery time. I have one of these machines and use it on minor injuries to lightly exercise the muscle without having to move the associated joints, it works for me on minor sprains and tears.

14. **STEROIDS.** These are known to dramatically increase anabolism and hence recovery ability, then there is hell to pay. Maybe not tomorrow, or even next month, but it will come back to haunt you and you will wish you hadn't taken them. Unless you have a doctors prescription they are illegal drugs and will be supplied by a drug dealer, with you having no idea what's actually in the bottle or file. Drug dealers will sell you anything to make money, please don't take illegal steroids.

15. **IBROFEN.** This is used to relive DOMS and is advertised as an anti-inflammatory drug. Some reports suggest an improved recovery, but it's inconclusive with several studies showing it's of no value in reducing DOMS or improving recovery. [*Br J Sports Med 1990*] Continued use can be damaging to the kidneys and cause intestinal bleeding. Leave it for when you're ill.

BLOCKERS

1. **STRESS.** Stress, whether at work or home is an enemy and can destroy your training as well as recovery. Stress could be caused by yourself, do your best to let things go, accept situations and look for practical win-win situations particularly in personal relationships. If the missus likes you to wash up do it before being asked with a smile. It's surprising how much more you receive from a little effort on your part. Happiness isn't a right, you have to earn it. Be realistic with expectations at work and home, 'so what' if you don't have a new car or have to work hard to pay the bills, that's life. Read a motivational book and try to get things into perspective, there are many people in this world who are far worse off than you, and you would do well to remember it!

2. **HANGOVERS**. Read and make sure you understand the section on the exercise hangover syndrome. Check your programme and change exercises or workout days to minimise or remove the elements causing the hangover. In particular, gain a better understanding of the muscles used in compound exercises and identify alternative exercises where necessary to reduce the multiple stress on muscles within your microcycle.

3. **INSULIN.** Insulin abuse is known to drive glycogen into muscle storage and is used in bodybuilding and other strength related sports. I hate to mention it, but it's out there. Silly people eat highly refined carbohydrate to raise their blood sugar then inject insulin to drive it into muscle storage. The side effects from getting it wrong are very serious and can kill you in one hit, don't do it.

4. **RECREATIONAL DRUGS.** These may make you feel totally up for it, but then the downside kicks in and it messes you up in just about every way. Only for dick heads!

5. **ALCOHOL.** In excess, this reduces anabolic liver functions while it's busy removing alcohol from the body and may extend your recovery time considerably. Ongoing excess reduces proper liver function and extends all recovery periods. However, one drink to help you relax after a hard session may actually provide some benefits. Use in moderation.

6. **SMOKING AND VAPING.** The poisons from smoking have to be eliminated from the body and will interfere with liver and kidney function. Smoking is totally counter productive and it will kill you, need I say more? Vaping, well, really?

7. **EXCESSIVE AEROBIC EXERCISE.** Aerobic exercise is important to maintain good heart and lung conditioning which helps local recovery, but the recovery requirements from excessive activity will delay or even stop strength development. If you can jog a mile comfortably that's enough, any more and your strength training will suffer.

Recovery is mainly common sense, a good protein rich, balanced diet with low impact active rest and a respect for your own body will help to minimise recovery time. You may be keen, and you may love going to the gym to workout, ok, if you want to train every day and socialise, fine! However, unless you've an excellent split routine you will be over training, and you won't make much progress. Understanding your own, or a trainees recovery needs is an important part of strength development planning and should be taken very seriously. As a personal example, some time ago I was struggling to improve a particular lift; it had stalled for months despite my efforts. My programme was sensible and the intensity was arranged in a 3-week wave, but my 3RM target was not improving at all. Then, through unexpected circumstances I couldn't do my usual Monday session and I eventually managed to get to the gym on the Wednesday. To my surprise, my strength was well above normal setting a new personal best 3RM, not once but for 5 sets on the trot, something that would have been unthinkable normally. This got me thinking about my own recovery periods. The seven-day period had worked well for years, but approaching 60 at the time I clearly needed longer. I extended my microcycle to 9 days for this particular exercise and the results were dramatic with personal bests being broken in the gym and at competition. I continued attending the gym on Mondays to coach, but kept my own programme running at 9 day intervals.

9. THE EFFECT OF GROWING STRENGTH ON RECOVERY TIMING

While any individual may grow in muscular weight very considerably over time with the right training, their internal organs that have to work hard to recover and replenish body functions don't. In fact, the recovery needs following intensive training will be extended as an individual grows.

When I started weight training as a fully grown young scroat at ten stone wet, I had virtually the same digestive system, liver and kidneys as I have now. However, now they are 50 years older and I've another 60 pounds of muscle to service 24 hours a day. It's simple math really, if my quadriceps have doubled in size, then intense strength training is likely to double the protein degradation as well as the local and systemic debt to recover. Consequently, my current recovery after a heavy session takes much longer than it used to. Now, at 72 years old I only train legs hard every 14 days, working a light 50% of 3RM one week without going to failure and heavy maximum 3RM the second on a rotation. I can't squat any more than 100kg because my sacra iliac joint likes to twist out, but I still use the 45% leg press. At 72 years old last week I pressed out 570kg for 3 repetitions from a right angled leg position. People in the gym assume I'm on loads of steroids, and several have asked what I'm taking, but I have never once touched them. I just train hard with the right recovery and nothing seems to stop me maintaining my strength.

Inevitably, if you continue to work to a high intensity to stimulate growth the additional muscle size and strength developed will require an ever increasing intensity of <u>training and recovery time</u> to continue the cycle. Some younger individuals will find their recovery time only increases a little due to improved muscle functions from long term training, but most trainees will need considerably more recovery time as they grow. Unfortunately, this concept is almost completely overlooked except in the most professional gyms and by well informed coaches. The story is very familiar in any gym you may visit. Beginners start with a typical three day a week programme and make good gains for a while, and then they reach a plateau. Why, because they are not recovering between workouts as their intensity has grown with their strength and muscle mass. Under recovery or over training has occurred. The graph in **Fig.14** shows the typical progress of a beginner to strength training over a year, measured by the combined weight of maximum singles in all the exercises used for a full body workout. It shows a beginner starting with three full body

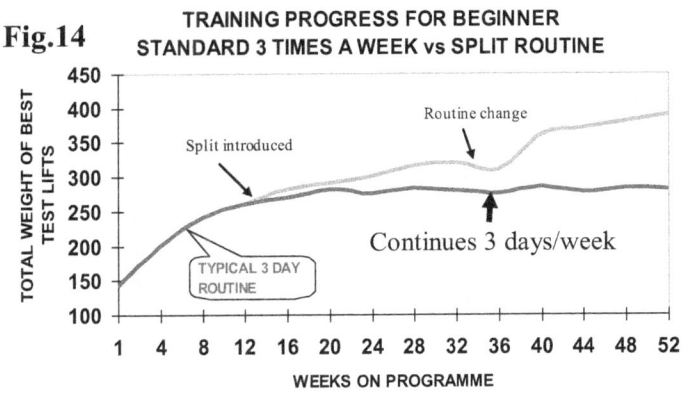

workouts a week at a low intensity, a popular starter programme. Initially good gains come from CNS improvements and muscle growth. However, after a while, improvements tail off as the intensity in each workout grows with increasing strength to a point where the recovery time in the programme is inadequate. At this point, unless the individual starts using a good split they will move into overtraining, and will fail to make progress as shown by the lower plateau line. Usually at this point all sorts of gym locker room advice kicks in, such as train more days, do negative sets, eat this, take that etc. Some advice may work for a while due simply to re-motivation, but then inevitably the whole programme fails, creating frustration. The programme must have more recovery time built in, and the easiest way to do this is with a split routine where body parts are trained separately and only once during a week, or microcycle. The graph upper line shows the result of introducing a split routine to train the main muscle groups only once a week over the same three days after 12 weeks. This allows each body part far longer to recover between training them again. A typical split may be; day 1, chest and shoulders, day 2, legs and back, day 3, arms and abdominals although there are countless other options. These three sessions may be spaced apart to suit the individual's recovery needs. Splits may be body parts, specialised exercises or competition preparation such as programmes for powerlifters based on the three lifts, typically day 1 squat and assistance work, day 2 bench press and assistance work and day 3 deadlift and assistance work. Later in the year the upper line shows a change in routine which initially results in a temporary worsening, followed by a strong return, and ongoing improvement. This is typical when introducing new exercises where the CNS has to learn to coordinate the movement, after which strong progress returns. The point I am making here, is that to progress over the long term you must increase the intensity <u>and</u> recovery time, <u>and</u> introduce variation regularly. As progress continues, the time between training sessions may need to be extended even farther. The 'wiser' coaches and trainees move the timing of workouts to ensure each one coincides with the super compensation phase to maintain ongoing development. Convincing a keen young trainee to do less is another story, particularly if they like the easy scheduled three days a week cycle and the social side of meeting others in the gym on regular days. Suggesting to a fired up powerlifter that to improve his stalled deadlift he must move to a 14 day rest period between sessions is like taking heroine from an addict.

While it may be unpopular, to make progress this is often the only solution to allow full recovery and avoid over training, potential injury and a continued stall in progress. You can alleviate the anxiety by introducing a 21 day, three week wave training pattern that only schedules one highly intense session for each of the three lifts every three weeks while training of some sort every week at a lower intensity.

Fig.15 shows a typical relationship between the intensity of muscle contractions required for ongoing development of the largest muscle groups, such as the quadriceps. For example, a beginner with a good coach may recover in five days from their leg workout when starting, but this may need extending by up to five days a year later after considerable growth and large strength increases. While this is not easily calculated for all individuals who vary considerably in recovery needs, as an individual grows in strength and experience the intensity of their training increases automatically **if they are training with any real intent**. Logically the recovery period has to increase correspondingly. High intensity training depletes body reserves very considerably, and very quickly. If you're doing large numbers of sets per body part, that training can't be at maximum intensity even if you're squealing like a stuck pig on the last rep. The most intense training involves very low repetitions of 3 or less with weights at 90% or more of T1RM, such as in powerlifting routines. Using near maximum weights for any exercise takes a huge effort both physically and mentally to complete, depleting the muscles and overall body reserves as well as the CNS capacity to cope with repeated demands. At my first British 3 lift championship I

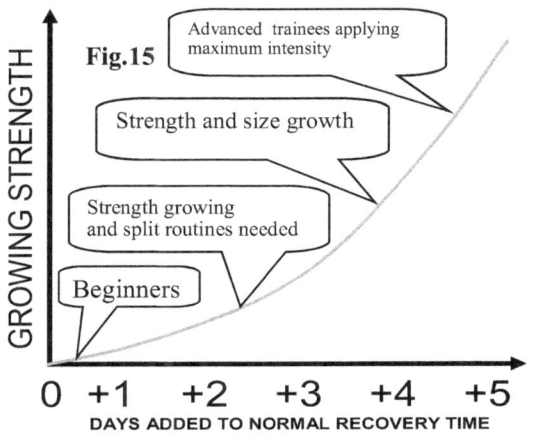

Fig.15

GROWING STRENGTH

Advanced trainees applying maximum intensity

Strength and size growth

Strength growing and split routines needed

Beginners

0 +1 +2 +3 +4 +5

DAYS ADDED TO NORMAL RECOVERY TIME

achieved my then personal best deadlift of 232.5kg in a competition. I was so pleased with myself that I decided to try it in the gym a week later. It appeared glued to the floor. I couldn't even get it to move apart from rolling it! I was so shocked I re-counted the weight thinking I had made a mistake. It took me nearly 3 weeks of active rest avoiding anything over 50% of T1RM for my deadlift to recover and get above 220kg again. Being over 55 years old at the time I should not have been surprised. The highest intensity training creates a massive drain on your body and even with the best nutrition and rest you will still need extended time to recover. Put bluntly, if you train again before recovery has taken place you're **WASTING YOUR TIME!** Yes, it's pointless and will drive recovery even farther away. Most gym users never really understand the relationship between intensity, recovery and growth in strength. I see trainees clattering away with multiple sets and multiple exercises per body part using relatively modest weights and never getting anywhere. Recently a young man asked me to help him improve his squat and general leg strength. I agreed to consider this if I could watch him train. He squatted first, which is always a good tactic, warming up with the empty bar he slowly progressing up to 100kg for 3 sets of 5 repetitions. He then went on to the 45 degree sledge leg press machine eventually ending with 3 sets of 8 with about 200kg. He was very pleased with himself and clearly thought he had impressed me. I smiled and said 'well done', then arranged to meet him the following week to coach him. He weighed about 95kg, and had been training for several years and had acquired a relatively good physique, but had been stuck for some months without progress. I could see just from his physique that 100kg on the squat was way below his capability, and 200kg on the leg press machine was ridiculously low for this young, healthy male. Talking to him after his workout, it was immediately apparent that he didn't have any specific goals and didn't record the results of any of his workouts. The following Monday, I met him to coach his workout. We started with the squat as normal and after several warm up sets he got to his 100kg working weight, at which point I said 'just do three repetitions' which he did with ease. He smiled and I could see he was thinking 'this is easy'. I then added 20kg to the bar for his next set, at which point he started to look a bit worried. 'Just do three repetitions instead of your usual 5', I said. With a little coaching on his breathing and technique he managed the three repetitions easily. At this point, I told him to get a drink and come back in five minutes while I put another 20kg on the bar. When he returned, he looked worried at the weight on the bar. I gave him plenty of encouragement and talked about the technique he should use while explaining exactly how I would be spotting him from behind and using the safety bars on the power rack. He did four repetitions to a good depth with the 140kg and with 5 minute rests he managed another two sets of four. Then we moved to the leg press machine. I let him warm up as usual, then after his first set at 200kg I added 40kg. With some encouragement he managed eight repetitions easily. I added another 40kg and he managed six repetitions. Another 40kg and another six repetitions. Another 40kg and a hard fought four repetitions. He repeated this 360kg for two more sets achieving four and three reps. He was now beginning to understand intensity and what you must do to move forward. The following week, after severe delayed onset muscle soreness lasting three days and another four days to recover and compensate he was ready for more. Armed with his new personal best results in a notebook I had given him, he was keen to beat them, and he did. This is just a simple example of accommodation to a routine; he was drifting without goals and without any real motivation or honest intensity. The application of authentic intensity and correct recovery drives growth in strength. Now, this growing lad has moved to a 14 day cycle and is fast approaching my weights!

10.   THE COMMON RECOVERY PATTERN

From numerous medical and sports research experiments a common recovery pattern has emerged. This applies to everyone, all ages, sexes, and experience levels. **Fig.16** shows how recovery happens over time following a single strength training event. The total recovery time needed to

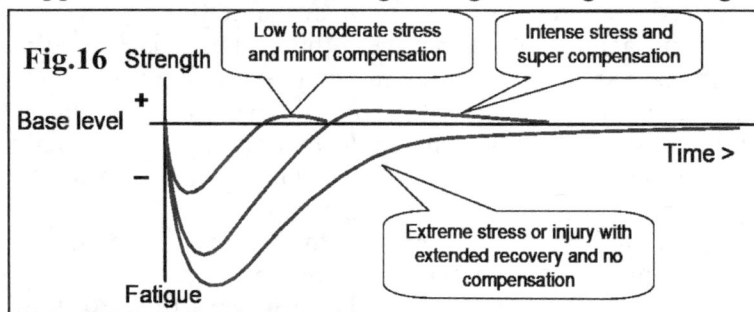

achieve the super compensation phase and normalisation of body chemicals and functions varies among individuals as already discussed. Consequently, the graph cannot accurately show any timescale due to the varying individual responses to exercise stress. The extreme stress line at the bottom of the graph shows how excessive muscular stress may result in extended recovery time and a complete lack of super compensation due to extensive damage, in real terms just getting back to the previous norm from high stress may be several weeks for some individuals.

The key to steady strength and muscular growth is the regular repetition of intense training at the correct interval within the super compensation phase. This drives a continuously improving strength capacity as indicated in **Fig.17**. The diagram represents the individual's strength, dropping after training events and recovering to super compensation before another training event. With this perfect sequence of training events within the super compensation periods continuous progress in strength and muscle size can be achieved.

Unfortunately, many trainees work the same muscles again before recovery or super compensation has occurred. If continued, serious over training fatigue develops resulting in the reverse process with declining strength and muscle capacity. **Fig.18** shows the effect of repeated stressful exercise on any muscles before recovery has taken place. This may be a direct result of deliberately training the same muscles too often, or the incorrect use of unsuitable compound exercises that inadvertently fatigue the same muscles in different sessions. The graphs shown are exaggerated for clarity, but the effects are clear in practice. Incorrect muscle stress timing will result in stalled progress, regression or even injury. This poorly planned incorrect sequencing of training generates severe local and systemic fatigue, which can be very debilitating requiring extended rest periods to get out of. For example, one powerlifter I knew had several crashes over an 18 month period where he experienced sudden drops in performance combined with a lack of enthusiasm to train,

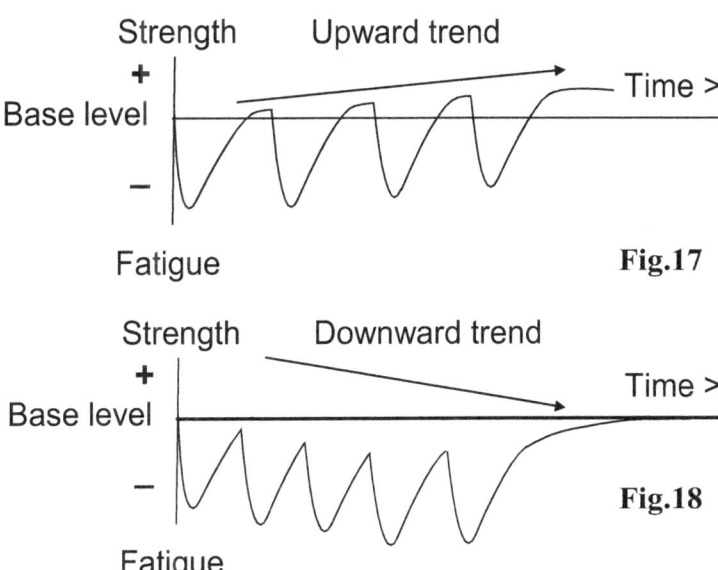

Fig.17

Fig.18

he even talked about giving it all up. During these times, he often caught a cold or throat infection and generally felt wrecked. When questioned, it was always the same issue; he'd driven himself too hard, training at the highest intensity every week without adequate rest. After 4-5 weeks of training with maximum weights he would hit the wall with his best lifts dropping by as much as 20%. After a de-load for a few weeks his strength miraculously returned. It was also noted that when he had a holiday, he returned renewed, determined and energetic, often producing his best results. This is a clear and observable pointer to over training resulting in chronic systemic fatigue. Multiple stress sessions may be used deliberately in a programme with careful planning of recovery as shown in **Fig.19**. Here a repeat intense training session is done after only a few days, driving the individual into greater fatigue, but followed by a lengthy recovery period. This is a

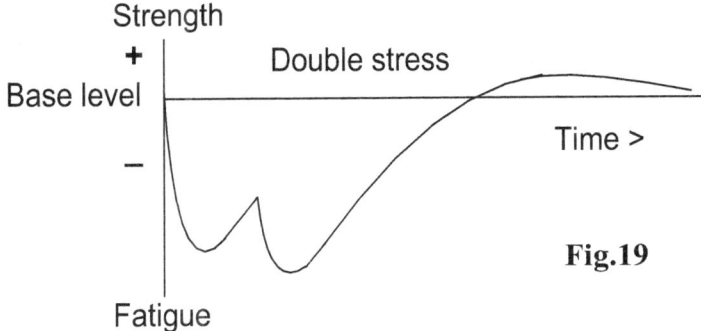

Fig.19

particularly useful device to use before a known break of several weeks such as a holiday where the normal run of training may result in the compensation phase being missed. This protocol may be increased to 3 intense sessions in a row with only a few days between them followed by 14 days or more rest.

I advise caution as such plans should be used very infrequently no more than twice in a season or year to avoid the possibility of injury. The recovery period is clearly longer, but may be planned to coincide with a return from a holiday or a special event or competition. Olympic lifters often use multiple sessions followed by relatively long rest periods before a major competition, although such methods have both mental and physical side affects which won't work for everyone. Some are stressed by the thoughts of a possible drop in performance before an event and it should be tried first for a holiday rather than a competition. Several lifters I have worked with seem to lose the mental capacity to work at 1RM after resting for more than a couple of weeks.

Athletes working at the top of their game are fragile, both physically and mentally and I always advise that finding what works for the individual rather than following a dogma is of paramount importance.

11. MULTIPLE SESSION RECOVERY ISSUES

The various graphs presented in the previous chapter mostly apply to single training sessions, for example, the medical study on the leg recovery of the 12 untrained men reaching super compensation in 7 days. The matter gets far more complicated with a full training programme where different muscles are stressed using a split routine.   From a single intense training session the capacity to recover is not overly stretched as the body may take as long as necessary. However, when sessions are stacked up over a short timescale the capacity of the body to systemically replete all the stressed muscles can become chronically exceeded.

The **systemic recovery deficit** is highly dependent on the training intensity and the size of the muscles exercised. As I have shown, the major leg muscle groups will require on average 7 days local and systemic recovery for fit young males following intensive stress, but individuals rarely leave it there. Recovery will be extended considerably if other exercise is undertaken in the recovery period. For example, if a trainee performs heavy squats and leg press on a Monday and they have excellent recovery capability they may expect to be fully recovered **and into super compensation** by the following Monday as indicated in **Fig.20, if they use good recovery protocols**.   However, what happens if they also train the bench press on Wednesday and

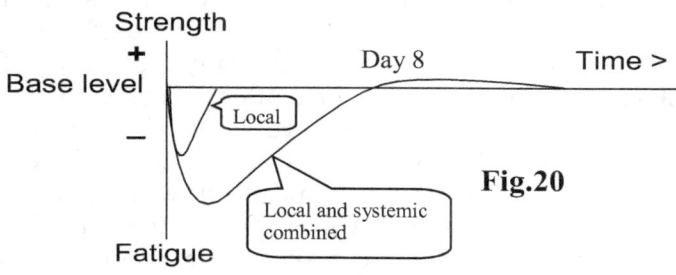

Fig.20

deadlifts on Friday? The systemic deficit will increase from each session. Systemic recovery relies on processes that take time and cannot be rushed, so the overall picture starts to become complicated as indicated in **Fig.21.** The cumulative affect of the systemic debt imposed on the body from this common three sessions a week powerlifting training has a massive impact on the body. You will note the bench press workout creates a lower systemic demand as the muscles involve are smaller, and require less systemic recovery. The deadlift session on the Friday makes a similar demand on systemic recovery to the squat. The consequences on strength

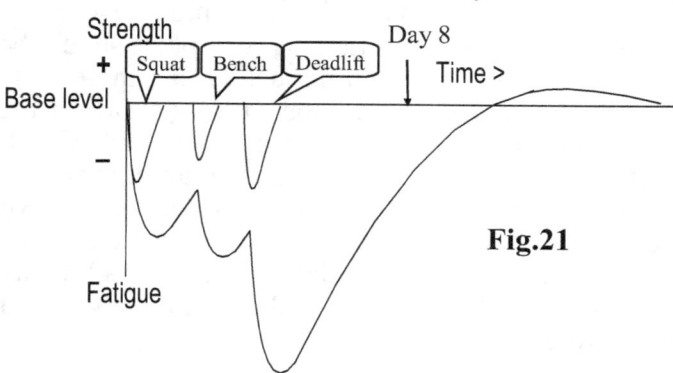

Fig.21

development are very significant, it could be 10 days before recovery is anywhere near super compensation for most of the muscles used. Without acknowledging this effect the powerlifter who continues to train at the maximum intensity three times every week will very soon reach a plateau, then if they continue with this plan their near maximum weights and 1RM performance will suffer. They are likely to experience minor muscle tears at best, or more serious injury at worst, along with mental anxiety from reduced performance. The solution for many lifters is a wave or step training pattern introducing periods of dynamic or lighter technique training between the highest intensity sessions for each exercise. Using this protocol allows full recovery over a longer period of two or three weeks before the next intense session on the same muscle group while still training weekly. An example plan is shown as **Fig.13** where each lift is only trained to 1RM intensity once every three weeks while still training weekly. **Fig.22** shows the effect of weekly intense squat sessions **in isolation** on a lifter who is failing to recover in 7 days. Here the lifter gradually moves into chronic fatigue from this over training. After several weeks, they are falling behind the curve and will experience drops in performance, a disinclination to train, and possible minor injuries. Unless additional recovery time is introduced into the plan as shown, performance will continue to deteriorate. Now, remember, this is for the squat in isolation, additional training makes the whole scenario far worse.

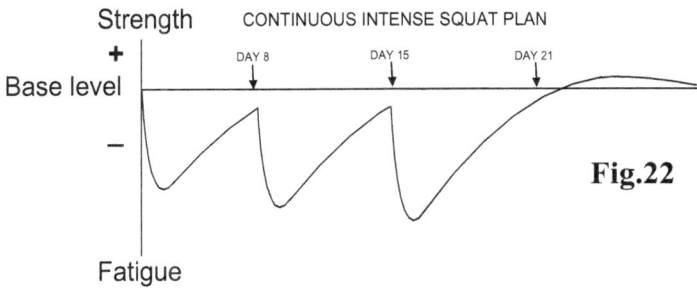

Fig.22

Solving this problem may be as simple as introducing a two step plan alternating intense sessions with technique training, such as, practising bar positioning, squat depth, foot positioning and the like, using only 50-60% of 1RM. The reduction in systemic fatigue from this sequence allows full recovery over a two week period as shown in **Fig.23.** This sequence of training will encourage the lifter giving them growing confidence from improved technical ability and performance. This is a simple example of how a step programme may provide an elegant solution that may be applied to any strength development plan. The lighter sessions may be aimed at correcting a technique deficiency, such as a poor depth on the squat, (powerlifter) or any targeted exercise that is not improving, the permutations are endless. Any exercise, sport or competition that needs technique work may be practiced in this way, and it's an ideal opportunity for trying a new style, (e.g. powerlifters trying the sumo stance for the deadlift) or positioning, such as grip and foot stance widths. Many experienced powerlifters also opt to use this lighter session for dynamic (speed) training to improve their rate of muscle motor unit recruitment.

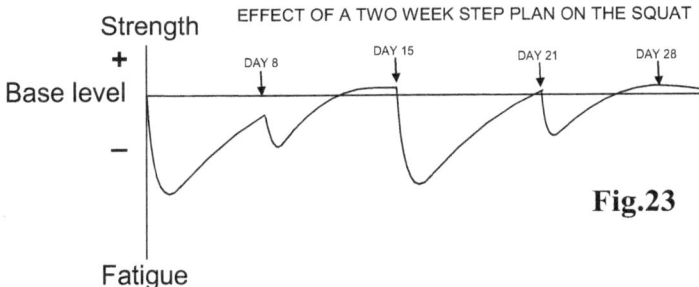

Fig.23

12. RECOVERY SUMMARY

We know that for pure strength and hypertrophy, improving muscle contraction capacity is important for continued progress. A lot may be achieved with CNS adaptation alone, but the limiting factor will always be the size, and hence contraction capacity of muscles used in a particular movement. Therefore, muscle size and conditioning are both important.

The recovery patterns shown in **Fig.16** are universal and have been reproduced from medical and sports studies across the world many times. This is accepted as fact, so please don't think that **you're** immune to this biological inevitability.

The elevated muscle contraction capacity available during the super compensation phase is exaggerated in the graphs for clarity. In reality, this is small, depending on the individual and the point in their training development. For beginners the picture gets complicated by large strength improvements from CNS adaptations. For hardened trainees getting the recovery period's right will result in a small improvement every microcycle. Typical improvements with experienced trainees may be as little as one additional repetition using a constant weight in a 3 set to failure plan for an exercise. Otherwise, a small 0.5-2.5kg increase in weight capability for 6 repetitions, but these figures will vary with individuals. Steady, small improvements are typical of the true nature of continuous strength gains once the beginners stage has been passed. Banking these small steps forward is the primary aim in strength training which add up over time. Apart from technique or dynamic training sessions a trainee should seek to make these small improvements at all intense workout sessions. If it's not forthcoming the first thing to consider is the recovery period since the last intense session. Recording performance is critical to this success as these small improvements may otherwise be lost. Record key target achievements to make any improvement or decline in performance visible. You need a clear signal if the recovery periods need adjusting.

At the other end of the scale inconsistency and long periods between training after the super compensation phase has elapsed, or failing to achieve a high enough intensity to stimulate compensation is under training taking the individual nowhere.

A note for coaches:
Over training or under recovery is a prevalent problem, particularly with novices who often wish to train every day or on set week nights with their mates in the gym.
Under recovery is not the same as over training, it's the result of appropriate strength training followed by other activity that interferes with recovery, typically sports such as football. Anyone attempting strength **and** sports training requiring a high element of endurance at the same time will encounter this problem. The body cannot develop both endurance and strength to any extent at the same time. Because of the nature of recovery from intense strength training it will be this element that becomes the loser.
Recently a young Latvian guy I was training for powerlifting made excellent progress right through the summer, then suddenly his progress stopped and his performance went into reverse. At the same time he lost 2kg in body weight over a three week period. Maybe you have guessed? It was the start of the football season and he played in a local team. Some trainees develop a social network through the gym and may do little else for male or female bonding, while others get a personal and emotional satisfaction from regular training with others. In addition, the endorphins released by the brain during and after intense exercise can create a feeling of pleasure that becomes addictive. All these issues may interfere with the training programme you may have planned with an individual. For example, you may specify a 6 or 8 day rest period between bouts of a particular exercise. Unfortunately, this means training on a different day each week which can 'ruin' the social aspect of meeting friends regularly on set days. Sometimes a coach may prescribe a 10-14 day rest between some exercises, but trainees may want to do more to meet their emotional needs due to the fear of 'losing touch' with the heavy weights. This urge to train intensely when recovery remains incomplete invites injury and a tendency to consider illegal steroids. As an individual you must seek to avoid it, and as a coach you must confront this early. Taking a hard line with a

complete ban on other gym work may prove to be unacceptable to the individual. One remedy is to suggest a trainee attends the gym on desired occasions to help mates with spotting, but to avoid any training themselves. Alternatively, the coach may set up a wave plan with light technique training following the highest intensity session. Whatever the solution the training plan must be adjusted to enable full recovery if the best results are to be gained.

The test of adequate recovery is really quite simple. If an exercise performed with the same weight at the same time in a subsequent workout does not produce a small improvement where all else is unchanged, then recovery is incomplete. It's as simple as that! In such cases a critical review of the time between training the same muscles must become a priority.
Extending the 7 day weekly cycle can be difficult for some, but don't be afraid of this, don't make excuses, just add one or two days to the normal recovery period before repeating the session. Find the right recovery time between repeat exercise and you will have the key to unlock progress.
There are many programmes aimed at allowing more regular training while recovery occurs, notably wave training with lower intensity sessions spaced between highly intense workouts designed for rate recruitment (dynamic) or technique training. Whatever you consider, now knowing how to look out for the problems will ensure you find a plan to suit you, or anyone you coach.

13. THE SPECIFIC ISSUE OF EXERCISE HANGOVERS

This section explains the hidden problem I call the '**exercise hangover syndrome**'. It's a problem present in strength and muscle building plans directly related to recovery that I find in nearly every workout I review, even with experienced lifters. It leads to a lack of progress, excessive DOMS and injuries.

Many exercises used to develop strength and hypertrophy are either badly sequenced or 'compound' in their generation of stress across several muscle groups, creating unsolicited stresses. The three powerlifting lifts are classic examples of compound exercises generating stress across multiple muscles. There is nothing wrong with that at all, as long as you're aware of the recovery issues they create. Often trainees use such compound exercises in a split sequence that compromises recovery. An example of this is the bench press. As a compound exercise it stresses the pectorals, triceps and anterior deltoids heavily, as well as impacting on the trapezius, latissimus and several lesser muscles around the shoulder blade at a lower intensity. Lets explore this example in a little detail.

If you train using the bench press or a similar machine exercise intensely to stress the pectorals they may be expected to recover inside 6-7 days as shown in **Fig.24**. However, the deltoids and triceps are also stressed needing to recover. Without further stress from other exercises, the deltoids will usually recover within 4-5 days as shown in **Fig.25**. I have ignored the stress on the triceps for the moment to make the explanation simpler, but the same issue will arise for the triceps. The actual recovery patterns depend on the training intensity, the grip width and the recovery capacity of the lifter, as well as the muscle balance between the major muscles used in this compound exercise. Some lifters with weaker pectorals find the anterior deltoids are more

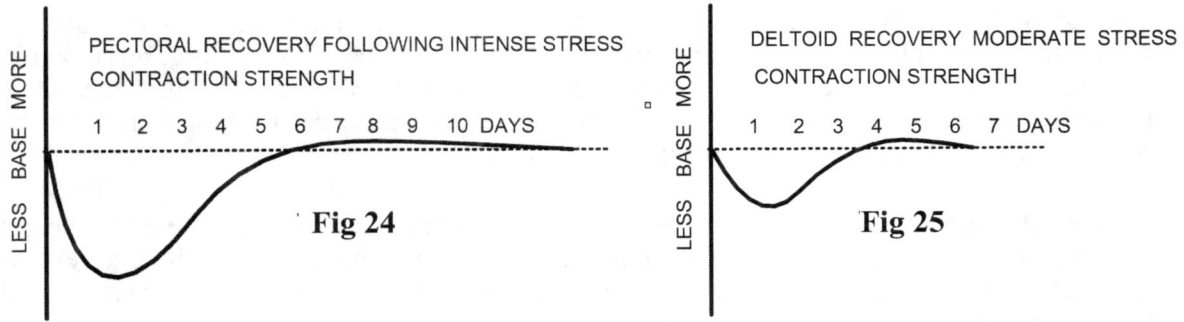

intensely stressed with the bench press. However, using typical average recovery figures, if nothing else stresses the pectorals before the next workout in 7 days (assuming a 7 day microcycle), they will gain strength steadily over the training cycles as shown in **Fig.26** reaching the point marked with a star after four weeks (day 29) where they are clearly stronger than the

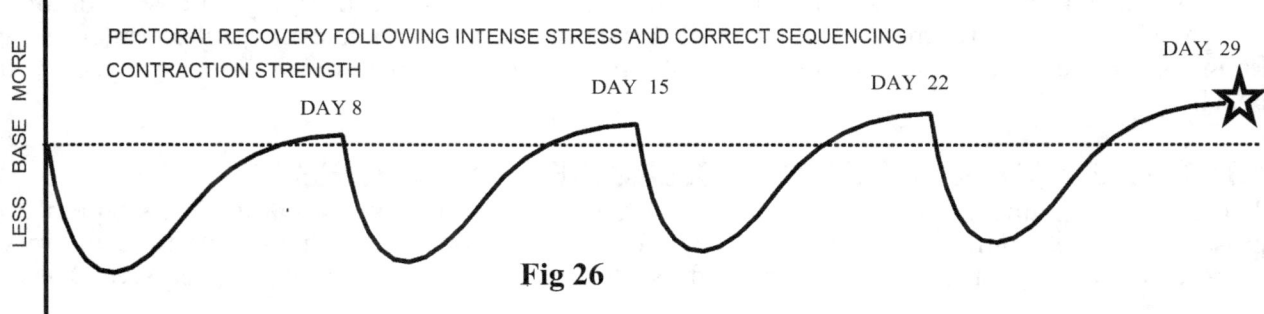

baseline at the start. But, what happens if the trainee decides to undertake a separate shoulder session every third day in the cycle? His deltoids would have reached super compensation in 4-5 days as shown in **Fig.25**, but on day 3 he trains them again with a separate shoulder workout. I have assumed the stress the anterior deltoid receives is similar to that from the bench press workout to simplify the example, but it could be far worse if the anterior deltoid stress is larger.

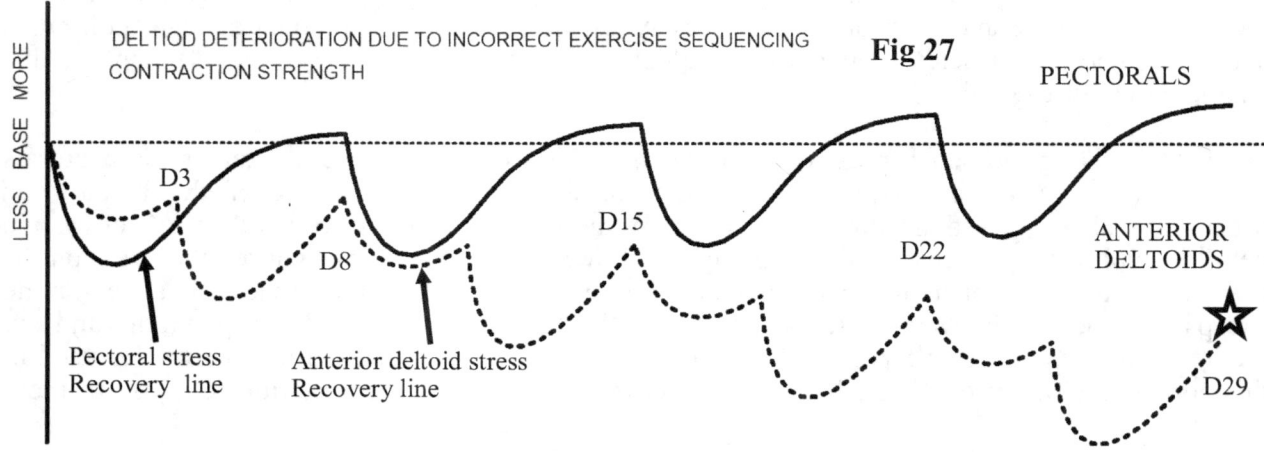

The repeated bench press workout on day 8, after a further 5 days stresses them again. This sequence of only 2 then 5 days rest for the anterior deltoids prevents them ever reaching recovery let alone super compensation and they descend into chronic over training as shown by the dotted line in **Fig.27**.   While the pectorals get stronger the deltoids are driven into chronic fatigue from training during a 'hangover' from previous un-recovered stress. This results in little progress on the bench press itself due to a lack of assistance from sore or possibly injured deltoids. The triceps will also encounter this problem if they are trained separately within the same 7 day microcycle.

I firmly believe that this scenario is a major contributing factor in many deltoid and shoulder injuries seen with competitive bench pressers. Note that the recovery days used in these examples are typical from very intense muscular stress, but will vary with intensity and individual recovery capability. On the other hand if you play with light weights this problem will most likely never occur and lack of progress will simply be down to a lack of appropriate intense stimulation.

Failure to understand the secondary effects on other muscle groups from compound exercises or bad sequencing will ruin any calculations for both local and systemic recovery. This is mitigated by training the multiple muscle groups involved on consecutive days, or virtually eliminated by training them on the same day. For instance, if you trained shoulders and chest on the same day using exercises that overlap in the use of similar muscles the recovery starts at the same time and assuming nothing else is stressing them in subsequent workouts the recovery will be fine. It's only when the same muscles are trained with different exercises more than 24 hours apart that the hangover starts to become a major issue.

Personally, I now train using two main programmes, either my whole upper body on one day and my legs and back on another in a 10 day microcycle, or Push, Pull, Legs alternating heavy and light weeks. Some powerlifters train the squat and deadlift on the same day, one at a high intensity and the other at a lower intensity using dynamic or technique training, they then invert this for the following microcycle. They do this because they have found it works quite well. The reason it works is because it minimises hangovers leaving the commonly used muscles a whole period of the training microcycle to recover and assuming good recovery a weekly microcycle may just work. With any split routine careful exercise selection is of prime importance. You must avoid any duplication of muscle group training which may result in extended recovery periods and a 'hangover' when performing subsequent sessions.

Coaches should watch out for this issue as hangovers have been present in just about every routine I've seen when reviewing new trainees existing plans. Powerlifters suffer more with hangovers as they often train the squat and deadlift weekly, severely stressing the quads, hams, spinal erectors and gluteus as well as calves twice every week. For powerlifters, avoiding lower back hangovers in particular may require a rotation plan with each primary lift only performed every 14, or even 21 days at the highest intensity. Watch out for hangovers in any suggested programme and question the design closely, you will be amazed how many otherwise excellent coaches fail to recognise this important training concept.

The next time someone suggests you do squats twice or more in a week, which seems to be a favourite on the internet, ask them how the legs will recover. Ask them about recovery times and the super-compensation cycle. I am betting they won't have a clue!

14.   CORRECTING A PROGRAMME WITH HANGOVERS

Hangovers are a constant source of frustration and injury, but you can dodge them with good planning and avoiding being coerced into joining your mates doing some crazy programme. It's a simple matter to estimate the recovery time of key muscle groups and adding them up over the repeated period of training (microcycle) to check for this systemic debt. As a rough guide the larger muscles of the legs have been scientifically demonstrated to need 7-9 days recovery from intensive work, while smaller muscles require less, typically 5-6 days for pectorals, triceps etc. Partial use in compound exercises, or from light to moderate sessions may be less than half these figures. In addition, it's important to remember that these figures are for fit, healthy young males. If you're not in this category, you may need to double or even treble these figures! Wow!

Has this made you think? It should.

Let's look at a typical example from a recent review that I undertook with a powerlifter. We discussed all the exercises he used in a seven day repeating microcycle and they are listed on **Fig.28.** He used a three session high intensity low repetition system for each exercise, and the

DAY	EXERCISE	pectorial	tricep	deltoid	traps	bicep	lats	quads	ham	calf	glutes	errectors	abs
	Microcycle of 7 days showing all exercises and estimated recovery periods in days												
DAY1	Bench press	6	4	4			2						
1	Tricep press		5									Fig.28	
1	Pec Deck	7											
1	Lat Pulls					3	6						
max recovery from day 1 required		7	5	4		3	6						
DAY 3	Deadlift				6	2		6	7	4	6	5	2
3	Shrugs				6								
3	Leg press							7	5	4	5		
3	Calf raise									5			
3	Low row					3	4					6	
max recovery from day 3 required				6	3	4	7	7	5	6	6	2	
DAY5	Squat							7	5	4	6	5	2
5	Crunch												5
5	leg Extension							7					
5	Bicep curl					5							
5	Upright row			5		2							
max recovery from day 5 required			5		5		7	5	4	6	5	5	
Total recovery required from cycle		7	5	9	6	11	10	14	12	9	12	11	7

likely recovery days are listed on the form. Where a muscle is stressed more than once by separate exercises on the same day only the highest recovery figure was used for that day. For example, on day 3 his calves generated a recovery debt of 4, 4 and 5 days respectively from deadlifts, leg press and calf raises, but only the highest figure of 5 is recorded for the day. This real example from a prominent gym surprised me. As I completed the assessment I became more and more animated seeing 8 muscle groups highlighted in bold were suffering from severe hangovers. I was horrified, and not surprised that the individual had asked for help. Those muscle groups showing over 7 days recovery needed were in a hungover state almost continually.

Note: the quads showing 14 days recovery required in a 7 day cycle!

This example shows how a poorly planned training programme can lead to severe over training of some muscle groups. Resolving it was relatively easy using the same exercises, but moving to a 21 day microcycle with the deadlift and squat sessions alternating between high and low intensity where the lower intensity sessions used dynamic and technique training. **Fig.29** shows this arrangement. You will see that both bench press sessions are at high intensity, this is possible as

DAY	EXERCISE	pectorial	tricep	deltoid	traps	bicep	lats	quads	ham	calf	glutes	errectors	abs
	Microcycle of 21 days showing all exercises and estimated recovery periods in days												
DAY1 load	Bench press	6	4	4			2						
1 load	Tricep press		5										
1 load	Pec Deck	7										**Fig.29**	
1 load	Lat Pulls					3	6						
max recovery from day 1 required		7	5	4		3	6						
DAY3 load	Deadlift				6	2		6	7	4	6	5	2
3 load	Shrugs				6								
3 load	Leg press							7	5	4	5		
3 load	Calf raise									5			
3 load	Low row					3	4					6	
max recovery from day 3 required					6	3	4	7	7	5	6	6	2
DAY7 de-load	Squat							3	3	2	3	3	1
7 de-load	Crunch												3
7 de-load	leg Extension							3					
7 de-load	Bicep curl					2							
7 de-load	Upright row			3		1							
max recovery from day 7 required				3		2		3	3	2	3	3	3
DAY10 load	Bench press	6	4	4			2						
10 load	Tricep press		5										
10 load	Pec Deck	7											
10 load	Lat Pulls					3	6						
max recovery from day 10 required		7	5	4		3	6						
DAY13 de-load	Deadlift				3	1		3	3	2	3	3	1
13 de-load	Shrugs				3								
13 de-load	Leg press							3	2	2	3		
13 de-load	Calf raise									3			
13 de-load	Low row					1	2					3	
max recovery from day 13 required					3	1	2	3	3	3	3	3	1
DAY17 load	Squat							7	5	4	6	5	2
17 load	Crunch												5
17 load	leg Extension							7					
17 load	Bicep curl					5							
17 load	Upright row			5		2							
max recovery from day 17 required				5		5		7	5	4	6	5	5
Total recovery required from cycle		14	10	16	9	17	18	20	18	14	18	17	11

the cycle being 21 days gave good recovery from both days. The new arrangement eliminated the hangovers with all muscle recovery totals less than 21 days. The individual started to make significant progress after only one cycle. The added advantage from this arrangement was variety in the workout, and the option to try different techniques such as the sumo squat in the light de-load sessions. As it happens, he liked the sumo squat and decided to use this method in competition which quickly improved his total. There were numerous other options to resolve the problem, but this particular arrangement suited the individual. He could have done the squat and deadlift on the same or subsequent days (within 24 hours) with a microcycle of 10 days as shown in **Fig.30** where all the muscles recover in less than the 10 day plan cycle. However, he thought

MICROCYCLE LENGTH	10	FORM TO ASSESS RECOVERY IN A TRAINING PROGRAMME

GUIDE TO RECOVERY REQUIRED IN DAYS FOR THOSE WITH GOOD RECOVERY CAPACITY

	pectorial	tricep	deltoid	traps	bicep	lats	quads	ham	calf	glutes	errectors	abs
HIGHLY INTENSE	6	6	6	7	5	7	8	7	5	5	7	5
MODERATE	4	4	4	5	4	5	6	5		4	5	4
LIGHT	3	3	3	4	3	4	4	4	3	3	4	3

DAY	EXERCISE	Intensity	pectorial	tricep	deltoid	traps	bicep	lats	quads	ham	calf	glutes	errectors	abs
1	squat	high							8	6	4	4	8	
1	leg extn	high	Fig.30						8					
1	calf mach	high									5			
1	deadlift	high				6	2	3	5	7	4	5	7	
1	low row	high				4	3	3	1	2	1	2	6	
1	tbar	high				2	3	5	1	1	1	2	5	
TOTAL FOR DAY 1						6	3	5	8	7	4	5	7	
2	bench p	high	6	5	5	3		3						
2	pec deck	high	6		3		1	2						
2	tri extn	high		6	2			2						
TOTAL FOR DAY 2			6	6	5	3	1	3						
TOTAL FOR MICROCYCLE			6	6	5	9	4	8	8	7	4	5	7	

that focussing on both the deadlift and the squat in the same session would be difficult. I agreed, have you ever worked both to maximum intensity on the same day? Not easy!

Alternatively, we could have dropped some assistance work and just extended the microcycle to fit. As you may appreciate there are many possible options. The point here is to show you how a plan is changed to eliminate hangovers, not to suggest the perfect plan. Whatever the option chosen, the results are often spectacular once the recovery between sessions has returned. This typical example is nothing unusual and not in any way exaggerated.

I recommend that you look closely at your own training plans, and consider the recovery of individual muscles that are inadvertently over trained from compound or poorly sequenced exercises and multiple sessions leaving a hangover. You might like to look at some plans advertised on the internet, they can be very amusing!

Remember, beginners are an exception as most of their gains in strength are from CNS adaptation and technique improvements. Beginners may show strength gains while actually over training with multiple hangovers, but this will soon catch them out.

Remove the hangovers, get the recovery right in any training programme and you have the recipe for progress, as long as diet, motivation, technique development and lifestyle are supportive, but that's another very, very long story for another time.

15. CHECKING TRAINING PROGRAMMES FOR HANGOVERS

The blank form at **Appendix A**, will enable you to check your training programme or any others for hangovers. Here's how to do it:

1. **Fill in the box at the top** for the microcycle length. This is the number of days a complete cycle of training plan takes. For example, if you have a simple 3 day a week plan then it will repeat on a 7 day cycle so enter 7. If on the other hand, you have a three week rotating wave pattern enter 21.

2. **List every exercise you perform** during each workout, even if you repeat an exercise in your microcycle on different days. You may for instance perform the bench press three times in a 21 day cycle at differing intensities, if so, enter the details three times. <u>Leave a clear line between separate day's workouts.</u>

3. **Enter the exercise intensity.** This dictates the recovery days you estimate for the primary and secondary muscles used in the exercises. Estimates are provided at the top of the form. If you think your recovery may be longer then provide your own estimates. DO NOT enter a shorter recovery than the guidance given as these figures are for fit, young, healthy males. Highly intense numbers are appropriate for extremely heavy low volume when performing maximum singles and doubles near or at 1RM or heavy multiple sets.

4. **Against each exercise listed, enter the recovery estimated** for ALL the major muscle used in the exercise. For example, for the deadlift enter a recovery estimate for; traps, erectors, hamstrings, calves, quadriceps and gluteus. Obviously, the primary muscles will be entered with the highest estimated recovery and the supporting muscles entered at around 50-75% of this figure. Some knowledge of the muscles used in compound exercises is required, if you're unsure ask an instructor or coach. Some guesswork on the relevant intensity for assisting muscles is inevitable, just be sensible.

5. **For each separate day's workout within your microcycle** select the highest individual recovery estimate for each muscle group where you have entered a figure, <u>do not add them up just use the highest number for that muscle group on that day.</u> Put these on the line you have left clear at the bottom for each day's session. If exercises with overlapping muscle usage are performed within 24 hours, for example if you train twice in one day you may record this as ONE DAY, but only once, if they are repeated again 24 hours later treat that as a separate day.

6. **Add up all the separate individual training day figures** for all the muscles, and enter these numbers on the total line at the bottom of the form.

7. **Those muscles with a total recovery number that is greater** than the microcycle length are almost certain to have a hangover from the training programme.

Removing the hangovers will require some thought and application of logic. The most obvious means to improve a training plan to remove them are:

1. **Extend** the microcycle length.
2. **Remove** some exercises, particularly assistance exercises in powerlifting training.
3. **Replace** compound with isolation exercises.
4. **Rotate** the intensity of some exercises, particularly those using the legs.
5. **Reduce** the volume of high intensity sets to lower systemic debt, then reduce recovery estimates for those muscles.

6. **Limit** or remove eccentric exercises and reduce recovery estimates.
7. **Use a wave** or step training pattern to introduce dynamic or technique sessions.
8. **Move exercises** that produce a large overlap of stress on common muscles to the same workout or within 24 hours of each other, then only use the highest recovery figure once in your calculations.

16 PLAN EXAMPLES

Before we look at a few examples of hangover free training plans I have to show you one that is on the Internet right now. This plan, written by a self proclaimed strength coach is one of the first on the google list on the web. It's a 3 day a week strength development plan with a 7 day microcycle. The exercises are as follows:

Monday	Wednesday	Friday
Squat	Front squat	Squat
Bench press	Military press	Bench press
T bar row	Pull up (chins)	Barbell row
Sit up	Curl	Bench Dips
Triceps extension	Crunch	Abdominal machine

Spot the problems yet? Well, you should by now have a good idea, and the first exercise on each day should worry you. If this were presented as a general fitness plan with high repetitions like an exercise class using light weights it would not be a huge problem at very low intensity. However, the plan suggests the squat should be performed using a 5x5 (five sets of five) where it's difficult to complete the last set of five repetitions. Depending on how hard this is worked it will generate a moderate or intense recovery situation. I'm going to be generous and assume the intensity is moderate. From this I have completed the recovery assessment as shown in **Fig.31** and not one muscle group will recover in a week, **not one**. For a beginner this may work for a few weeks as they develop CNS coordination and make some strength gains despite the growing systemic fatigue, for anyone else it's a disaster. What more can I say?

There are many more like this published by people who should know better, and you would do well to steer clear of such crap. Now, I'm trying not to be cynical, but everyone and their dog seem to think a few months in a gym makes them an expert. It doesn't. General fitness is not strength training, if you want to get strong you need to super compensate! Let's put all that negativity to one side and look at some good hangover free plans that will work for most trainees with average recovery capacity.

Example 1. Fig.33 shows an example for a general all body strength plan that can be done on a simple 7 day cycle with three workouts indefinitely, until you need to change some exercises for variety. It uses the working weight system with three working sets. After a general body warmup and a light warm up for each exercise the three working sets are done with 3 minute rests between the working sets. Each set is taken to muscle failure and the repetitions achieved in total are targeted at 24 before raising the weight for the next week. When bodyweight exercises (chins and sit up) hit target, add weight with a weight belt or holding a disc. You will note that there are only

MICROCYCLE LENGTH			7	FORM TO ASSESS RECOVERY IN A TRAINING PROGRAMME										
GUIDE TO RECOVERY REQUIRED IN DAYS FOR THOSE WITH GOOD RECOVERY CAPACITY														
HIGHLY INTENSE			6	6	6	7	5	7	8	7	5	5	7	5
MODERATE			4	4	4	5	4	5	6	5	4	4	5	4
LIGHT			3	3	3	4	3	4	4	4	3	3	4	3
DAY	EXERCISE	Intensity	pectoral	tricep	deltoid	traps	bicep	lats	quads	ham	calf	glutes	errectors	abs
1	squat	moderate							6	5	3	3	5	
1	bench pr	moderate	4	4	4									
1	bar row	moderate				3	3	5						
1	sit up	moderate												4
1	tri extn	moderate		4										
TOTAL FOR DAY 1			4	4	4	3	3	5	6	5	3	3	5	4
2	front squat	moderate							5	4	3	3	3	
2	mil press	moderate		3	4	3								
2	deadlift	moderate				4		3	5	5	3		5	
2	chin	moderate					4	4						
2	curl	moderate					4							
2	crunch	moderate												4
TOTAL FOR DAY 2				3	4	4	4	4	5	5	3	3	5	4
3	squat	moderate							6	5	3	3	5	
3	bench pr	moderate	4	4	4									
3	bar row	moderate				3	3	5						
3	dips	moderate		4			2	4						
3	abs mach	moderate												4
TOTAL FOR DAY 3			4	4	4	3	3	5	6	5	3	3	5	4
TOTAL MICROCYCLE RECOVERY			8	11	12	10	10	14	17	15	9	9	15	12

Fig.31

Example of a bad plan recovery analysis.

WTF?

four exercises per workout and with a good 3 minutes rest between working sets the sessions will be done in an hour. Due to the relative high number of repetitions, the intensity even when pushed hard will only amount to a moderate recovery requirement. You should note that all body parts will be in the super compensation phase within the 7 day cycle. Don't do anything else in the gym other than some light recovery work. This plan will lead to excellent strength gains.

Example 2. Fig.34 Shows an example powerlifting plan that won't leave you with a hangover. It's based on a 14 day rotation with three workouts in each of the two weeks. The squat and deadlift are performed at alternating high and low intensity one day in each week with the bench press having a high intensity one week and a low intensity the other. There are several assistance exercises included with no more than three exercises in total for each workout. The squat and deadlift high intensity sessions should be performed for the best 3 repetition weights using a 3 and up process and high intensity assistance exercises at 6up. 3up means starting at a moderate weight for three reps only, adding weight and doing another 3 reps after 3 minute rest periods until 3 reps becomes impossible, 6up follows the same process using 6 repetitions. 1RM tests are added to the high intensity sessions every 4th session for the three powerlifting exercises only. On 1RM days you may completely leave out the assistance work. The low intensity squat and deadlift sessions should be done with 50% 1RM weights for three sets of 12 regardless of capability, do not go to failure and use dynamic effort for the deadlift and technique training for both. For example, the squat may be trained to just lower than thighs parallel to the floor when performing

MICROCYCLE LENGTH		7	FORM TO ASSESS RECOVERY IN A TRAINING PROGRAMME											
GUIDE TO RECOVERY REQUIRED IN DAYS FOR THOSE WITH GOOD RECOVERY CAPACITY														
HIGHLY INTENSE			6	6	6	7	5	7	8	7	5	5	7	5
MODERATE			4	4	4	5	4	5	6	5	4	4	5	4
LIGHT			3	3	3	4	3	4	4	4	3	3	4	3
DAY	EXERCISE	Intensity	pectoral	tricep	deltoid	traps	bicep	lats	quads	ham	calf	glutes	errectors	abs
1	leg press	moderate							6	5	4	4		
1	calf raise	moderate									4			
1	leg exten	moderate							6					
1	sit up	moderate												4
TOTAL FOR DAY 1									6	5	4	4		4
2	db lat raise	moderate				4	2							
2	bench pres	moderate	4	4	4		2	1						
2	tricep ext	moderate			4									
2	pec deck	moderate	4											
TOTAL FOR DAY 2			4	4	4	4	2	1						
3	bar shrugs	moderate			2	5	2							
3	cable curl	moderate				2	4							
3	bw chins	moderate					2	5						
3	hyper extn	moderate				3	2	2					5	
TOTAL FOR DAY 3					2	5	4	5					5	
TOTAL MICROCYCLE RECOVERY			4	4	6	6	4	6	6	5	4	4	5	4

Fig.33
General all body plan for a 7 day cycle recovery analysis

low intensity to embed the feeling of depth for when the high intensity sessions are undertaken. All the other exercises should be performed with 50% of 1RM for low intensity sessions and 75% of 1RM for moderate intensity sessions. For both these intensities don't go to full muscle failure. This plan will work very well for most individuals with moderate to good recovery capability, nevertheless if your squat and deadlift results are poor you may need more recovery and extending the plan to 16 days should resolve the issue. The weights will tell you if its working so be sure to record your 3up and 1RM weights.

Example 3.   Fig.35 shows a plan intended for competitive powerlifters who compete exclusively in the equipped bench press wearing bench press shirts. It's based on a 14 day microcycle with two sessions a week building on technique to peak with a 1RM session in day 4. The sessions should be several days apart, typically Monday and Thursday.

Day one is a raw (no shirt) bench press day using sets of 5 at 75-80% of R1RM, followed by a highly intense triceps 3 up session and a moderate 12 up pectoral session on the Pec deck .

Day two is a session where only light bench weights of 50% of R1RM are used to practice arching the back using foam or pads. This is an ideal time to practice dynamic pressing. This is followed by an intensive abdominal 6up and lower back session using hyperextensions holding a disc for 12up. The objective of day 2 is to strengthen and improve the core and arching capability.

Day 3 is a session to practice positioning and arching wearing the bench press shirt at a low intensity. Most bench shirts if correctly fitted won't allow the bar to touch the chest with 50% E1RM and it's advisable to use wooden blocks on the chest while practicing the arch wearing the shirt. Ensure you have safety bars on the bench and competent spotters.

This is followed by a low intensity triceps extension session using 3 sets at 50% of previous 3up

MICROCYCLE LENGTH		14	FORM TO ASSESS RECOVERY IN A TRAINING PROGRAMME											
GUIDE TO RECOVERY REQUIRED IN DAYS FOR THOSE WITH GOOD RECOVERY CAPACITY															
HIGHLY INTENSE			6	6	6	7	5	7	8	7	5	5	7	5
MODERATE			4	4	4	5	4	5	6	5	4	4	5	4
LIGHT			3	3	3	4	3	4	4	4	3	3	4	3
DAY	EXERCISE	Intensity	pectoral	tricep	deltoid	traps	bicep	lats	quads	ham	calf	glutes	errectors	abs
1	squat	high							8	7	5	5	5	
1	deadlift	low				2			4	4	3	3	4	
1	leg exten	moderate							6					
TOTAL FOR DAY 1						2			8	7	5	5	5	
2	bench pres	low	3	3	2	1		1						
2	tricep ext	low		3										
2	pec deck	low	3											
TOTAL FOR DAY 2			3	3	2	1		1						
3	ab mach	high												5
3	bw chins	moderate					4	5						
3	bench dec	low	3	3	2	1		2						
TOTAL FOR DAY 3			3	3	2	1	4	5						5
4	squat	low							4	4	3	3	3	
4	deadlift	high				7			6	7	4	5	7	
4	leg exten	low							4					
TOTAL FOR DAY 4						7			6	7	4	5	7	
5	bench pres	high	6	6	6	2		2						
5	tricep ext	moderate		4										
5	pec deck	moderate	4											
TOTAL FOR DAY 5			6	6	6	2		2						
6	db lateral	moderate			4									
6	bw chins	moderate					3	4						
6	t bar row	moderate					4	5					1	
TOTAL FOR DAY 6					4		4	5					1	
TOTAL RECOVERY			12	12	14	13	8	13	14	14	9	10	13	5

Fig.34
Powerlifting plan without hangovers recovery analysis

and a low intensity pectoral stretching session **using light dumbbells** for fly allowing the pectorals to stretch out.

Day four is the highly intense session on the bench wearing the competition bench press shirt and doing singles. Warm up raw with doubles and singles, then at around 60-75% of E1RM put on the bench shirt and start doing singles to competition standards, i.e. with a pause on the chest. Take five minutes between singles when over 75% of E1RM and ensure you have safety bars and competent spotters. This is followed with light stretching work for the abdominals and erectors.

The examples above are intended to show you clearly how a strength programme may be put together in such ways to ensure you repeat your training with your body in the super compensation phase within every microcycle. I have waived the copyright to appendix A, so you may copy it for your own use as much as you like.

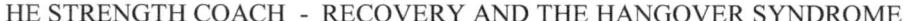

MICROCYCLE LENGTH		14	FORM TO ASSESS RECOVERY IN A TRAINING PROGRAMME											
GUIDE TO RECOVERY REQUIRED IN DAYS FOR THOSE WITH GOOD RECOVERY CAPACITY															
HIGHLY INTENSE			6	6	6	7	5	7	8	7	5	5	7	5
MODERATE			4	4	4	5	4	5	6	5	4	4	5	4
LIGHT			3	3	3	4	3	4	4	4	3	3	4	3
DAY	EXERCISE	Intensity	pectorial	tricep	deltoid	traps	bicep	lats	quads	ham	calf	glutes	errectors	abs
1	bench pres	mod Raw	4	4	3	2		1						
1	tricep ext	high		6										
1	pec deck	mod	4											
TOTAL FOR DAY 1			4	6	3	2		1						
2	bench pres	arch Raw	1	1	1	1		1					3	
2	abs mach	high												5
2	hyper extn	high											7	
TOTAL FOR DAY 2			1	1	1	1		1					7	5
3	bench pres	low arch E	3	3	3	2		1					2	
3	tricep ext	low		3										
3	pec deck	stretch	3											
TOTAL FOR DAY 3			3	3	3	2		1					2	
4	bench pres	max Equipt	6	4	4	5		5						
4	abs mach	light stretch												1
4	hyper extn	low arch											4	
TOTAL FOR DAY 4			6	4	4	5		5					4	3
TOTAL RECOVERY			14	14	11	10	0	8	0	0	0	0	13	8

Fig.35
Bench press powerlifting recovery analysis

Finally, remember that all the information given in this booklet is backed by medical science for clean drug free athletes. A great deal more is available on several key medical publications sites like 'PubMed', have a look and see for yourself how science backs up everything I have written about in this booklet. Perhaps more importantly, my comments are borne out from over 55 years of practical experience and proven to me on many occasions to be accurate and relevant to anyone who trains with weights to get stronger. The information in this booklet will set you on the path to gains in strength and muscular capacity that you may have thought impossible without drugs. You <u>can</u> do it the right way! Will you? Won't you? Well, that's up to you.

If in doubt, <u>do less</u>, it could make all the difference to your progress.

Now it's up to you, good luck!

NOTES:

MICROCYCLE LENGTH		FORM TO ASSESS RECOVERY IN A TRAINING PROGRAMME												
GUIDE TO RECOVERY REQUIRED IN DAYS FOR THOSE WITH GOOD RECOVERY CAPACITY														
HIGHLY INTENSE		6	6	6	7	5	7	8	7	5	5	7	5	
MODERATE		4	4	4	5	4	5	6	5	4	4	5	4	
LIGHT		3	3	3	4	3	4	4	4	3	3	4	3	
DAY	EXERCISE	Intensity	pectorial	tricep	deltoid	traps	bicep	lats	quads	ham	calf	glutes	errectors	abs
TOTAL RECOVERY														

NOTES:

ABBREVIATIONS AND GLOSSARY OF UNUSUAL TECHNICAL TERMS

ACCOMMODATION	The development of staleness from repeated use of the same routine over extended periods.
ASSISTANCE EXERCISE	An exercise that helps develop the muscles used in a primary movement or competitive lift.
ASYNCRONIOUS	The recruitment of muscle motor units in a shared serial manner.
BOMB	Failing all three attempts of one lift in a competition and being disqualified.
C1RM	The maximum single lift weight achieved in competition.
CNS	Central Nervous System. The brain and spinal cord and associated nervous system.
COMPOUND EXERCISE	An exercise that employs multiple muscles across one or more joints in the skeleton.
CYCLIC	A training plan that has a repeating pattern over sequential sessions.
DOMS	Delayed onset muscle soreness. Stiffness and ache usually 24-48 hours after intense training.
DYNAMIC EFFORT	Repetitions performed for speed development of motor unit recruitment, usually with 50-60% of 1RM weight.
EQUIPPED	Bench press, squat or deadlift wearing a bench shirt or powerlifting body suit.
E1RM	Equipped maximum single lift.
FORCE VELOCITY DEFICIT	The time lag between the execution of a movement and the application of maximum contraction in the muscles.
GBPF	Great Britain powerlifting Federation. The primary IPF affiliated organisation in the UK.
HANGOVER	An unplanned fatigue in one or more muscles remaining from additional sessions between key exercise sessions.
IPF	International powerlifting Federation, the leading world organisation for powerlifting.
HANG	The bar held above the chest by the tension in a bench shirt.
HOMEOSTASIS	The normal fully recovered status of the body or muscle.
LATS	Latissimus Dorsi, the large muscles of the back giving the inverted triangle shape.
MAXIMAL EFFORT	A set where only one single repetition is possible.
MICROCYCLE	A complete single cycle of training, often a week or ten days in a training plan.
MESOCYCLE	A group of micro-cycles, often a month in a training plan.
PB	Personal best performance.
PDCAAS	Protein digestibility corrected amino acid score. The measure of protein quality for human tissue balance.
PEC	Pectoral chest muscle.
R1RM	Unequipped (raw) maximum single lift.
RAW	Bench press, squat or deadlift without a bench shirt or powerlifting body suit.
RECRUITMENT RATE	The speed at which muscle motor units are fired following the conscious decision to contract.
REPEATED EFFORT	A set where repetitions are taken to muscular failure.
STATIC CONTRACTION	The performance of an exercise statically against great resistance.
SUB-MAXIMAL EFFORT	A set where repetitions are stopped before muscular failure.
SUPER COMPENSATION	The increase in muscle capability once recovery has been completed.
SYNCRONIOUS	The recruitment of muscle motor units together in parallel.
SYNERGIST	A supporting or holding muscle, contracting to hold a body position.
TETANUS	The full fusing of a muscle under maximum contraction.
T1RM	As for 1RM but limited to training in the gym.
VAL SALVA	Holding the breath while exercising, usually with a compression of the chest.
1RM	One rep maximum. The maximum weight capable of being performed for one single repetition.

REFERENCES AND USEFUL SOURCES

GBPF	http://www.gbpf.org.uk/
HAMILTONS	http://www.hamiltonsfitness.co.uk/weightlifting.htm
ENGLISH POWERLIFTING	http://www.englishpowerlifting.co.uk/
BDFPF	http://www.bdfpa.co.uk/
IPF	http://www.powerlifting-ipf.com/
PULLUM SPORTS SUPPLY	http://www.pullum-sports.co.uk/
SUGDEN FORUM	http://www.sugdenbarbell.co.uk/forum

ACKNOWLEDGEMENTS

My special thanks to James, John, Dan, Edwardo and Mason for their known and unknown contribution to this booklet as guinea pigs.

My thanks to Mark Cotton and Martin Green for putting up with all the noise and chalk in their gyms.

My thanks to Cathy and Stuart of Hamiltons in Colchester for getting me started in powerlifting.

My thanks to Mike Vernon for showing me the way and putting me on the right path for life.

A special thanks to my wife Lynda for putting up with all the undone work that built up while I was writing this booklet!

For more information on the science behind muscle strength development, training techniques and specific detailed information on developing the three powerlifting movements of the Squat, Bench Press and Deadlift, as well as Coaching and Motivating techniques see:

THE STRENGTH COACH - DEVELOPING THE BENCH PRESS

THE STRENGTH COACH - TRAINING TECHNIQUES AND METHODS

THE STRENGTH COACH - COACHING AND MOTIVATING POWERLIFTERS

THE STRENGTH COACH - THE KEYS TO SUCCESSFUL STRENGTH TRAINING